INSIDE DOCTORING

INSIDE DOCTORING

Stages and Outcomes
in the Professional Development
of Physicians

Edited by

Robert H. Coombs, Ph.D.,
D. Scott May, M.D.,
and Gary W. Small, M.D.

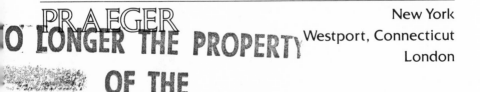

PRAEGER

New York
Westport, Connecticut
London

Library of Congress Cataloging-in-Publication Data

Inside doctoring.

  Includes bibliographies and index.
  1. Medicine – Vocational guidance.
2. Physicians – Mental health. 3. Professional
socialization. I. Coombs, Robert H. II. May,
D. Scott. III. Small, Gary W. [DNLM:
1. Education, Medical. 2. Physicians.
3. Physician's Role. W 21 I59]
R690.I56 1986   610.69'52   86-15083
ISBN 0-275-92172-7 (alk. paper)
ISBN 0-275-92173-5 (pbk. : alk. paper)

Library of Congress Catalog Card Number: 86-15083
ISBN: 0-275-92172-7
ISBN: 0-275-92173-5

First published in 1986

Praeger Publishers, 521 Fifth Avenue, New York, NY 10175
A division of Greenwood Press, Inc.

Printed in the United States of America

The paper used in this book complies with the Permanent
Paper Standard issued by the National Information Standards
Organization (Z39.48-1984).

10 9 8 7 6 5 4 3 2 1

Acknowledgments

We gratefully acknowledge the contributions of our students, particularly Michelle Beshara and Jeffrey Young, who contributed substantially to this effort. We also express appreciation to Carla Cronkhite and Karen Moody, who skillfully handled administrative details, and to Michael Fisher, Medical Editor at Praeger, whose thoughtful criticism improved the book's focus and quality.

We acknowledge with appreciation the authors and publishers who have allowed us to print or reprint their materials. For those publications reprinted here, we gratefully acknowledge:

Daniel Bressler, "Notes from Overground: Fourth Year at Harvard Medical School," *Journal of the American Medical Association*, Vol. 245, No. 16, April 24, 1981, pp. 1637–1638. Reprinted by permission of the *Journal of the American Medical Association*. Copyright 1981, American Medical Association.

Anonymous, "The Chief," *Journal of the American Medical Association*, Vol. 246, No. 13, September 25, 1981, pp. 1457–1458. Reprinted by permission of the *Journal of the American Medical Association*. Copyright 1981, American Medical Association.

Norman Cousins, "Internship: Preparation or Hazing?" *Journal of the American Medical Association*, Vol. 245, No. 4, January 23/30, 1981, p. 377; "Internship: Physicians Respond to Norman Cousins," *Journal of the American Medical Association*, Vol. 246, No. 19, November 13, 1981, pp. 2141–2143; "Norman Cousins Responds," *Journal of the American Medical Association*, Vol. 246, No. 19, November 13, 1981, p. 2144. Reprinted by permission of the *Journal of the American Medical Association*. Copyright 1981, American Medical Association.

Gary W. Small, "House Officer Stress Syndrome," *Psychosomatics*, Vol. 22, No. 10, October 1981, pp. 860–864. Reprinted by permission of the *Journal of the Academy of Psychosomatic Medicine*. Copyright 1981, The Academy of Psychosomatic Medicine.

Anonymous, "The Goal," *Journal of the American Medical Association*, Vol. 250, No. 3, July 15, 1983, p. 407. Reprinted by permission of the *Journal of the American Medical Association*. Copyright 1983, American Medical Association.

Suzanne Trupin, "When the Obstetrician Gets Pregnant," *MEDICA: Women Practicing Medicine*, Vol. 2, No. 1, February 1984, pp. 103–104. Reprinted by permission of *MEDICA: Women Practicing Medicine*. Copyright, 1981.

John J. Secondi, "A Short Guide to Doctors," *Journal of Irreproducible Results*,

Preface

Medical dramas are inherently interesting; the universal plot, a struggle against death and disease, compellingly concerns all mankind. In all societies, through each generation of time, those cast in the role of healers, with real or imagined powers over these ubiquitous enemies, have been held in highest respect, sometimes even regarded with worshipful reverence.

In American society, physicians have also been a source of considerable public fascination. Few, if any other careers have captured the interest and imagination of so many. Each breakthrough in medical science and technology has added additional luster to the physician's image.

Capitalizing on public interest in medical matters, the mass media have heightened popular interest and contributed further to the physician's mystique. With such glamorous portrayals, is it any wonder that so many young people aspire to medical careers, often from their early childhood? Who wouldn't want to live the exciting medical lifestyle or become like the warm, sensitive physicians portrayed in television dramas?

Imbued with romanticized conceptions of the physician's status and role, actual exposure to the physicians' inner sanctum can be a jarring experience. Entering medical students, possessed of popularized notions, are often shocked when confronted with these realities. Despite years of rigorous work to gain admission, many first-year medical students consider the possibility of withdrawing— four out of ten in one study.* Although very few actually drop out, a sense of disillusionment and resentment occurs often. This attests to the considerable gap between popularized notions and the realities of the medical milieu.

Alas, physicians are only mortal and subject to the same vicissitudes and degenerative processes that affect us all. Offstage and on, they too experience the full range of human problems and emotions. But this aspect of their existence is generally hidden to all

---

*Robert H. Coombs. *Mastering Medicine: Professional Socialization in Medical School.* New York: The Free Press, Macmillan Publishing Company, 1978.

but those who share their world. And more often than not, very little sharing of personal feelings occurs between them. Despite high stress and constantly challenging circumstances, emotional isolation is all too typical.

It has been our opportunity to participate intimately in this world. Two of us (May and Small) have personally survived the demanding processes of medical training and are now practicing physicians. Another (Coombs) has for two decades, as a Professor of Medical Sociology at two medical schools, made "doctor watching" (research and teaching on this topic plus private counseling with medical trainees and practitioners) one of his primary professional activities. The three of us share a common fascination with the social and psychological processes that shape young men and women into societally sanctioned healers. Our main interest is in understanding the personal struggles and adjustments required of those who gradually embrace this demanding role.

The aim of this book is to provide a behind-the-scenes account of the physician's private domain. A search for insightful writings about the physician's experience has occupied more than four years of effort. Students who have taken our UCLA course, "Professional Socialization in the Physician's Career," have, with us, spent hundreds of hours culling through the literature searching for printed narratives that capture a feeling for what it is like to be a physician, to routinely deal with many of life's most challenging and poignant circumstances. Our purpose has been to locate and select writings that are informative and interesting and provide a *verstehen*, an insider's grasp of reality. This book is the outcome of these efforts.

The book is designed for courses like our own courses for pre-medical students, first-year medical students, and/or medical couples. For this reason, lists of additional reading are included with each chapter. Our hope is that such courses will soon become regular offerings at every medical school and each undergraduate college that enrolls prospective physicians. We have learned from several years' experience that class discussions are consistently provocative and personally beneficial when based upon stimulating reading materials and reinforced by appropriate videotapes and expert discussants (medical students and physicians of varying stages and circumstances, spouses, patients, etc.). When, in addition, arrangements are made for students to interact regularly with a physician preceptor, a clear grasp of medical realities is gained and later disillusionment avoided.

We have organized the book into two parts. The first section traces the evolution of doctors through the sequential stages of training and practice—undergraduate "pre-med" training, medical school, internship, residency, fellowship, medical practice, and retirement. The second section focuses on potential developmental outcomes that may result: emotionally impaired doctors are contrasted with "compleat" physicians, those who have integrated in a balanced manner the emotional with the intellectual and technical aspects of their careers.

We wish that all medical trainees could become "compleat" physicians, and hope that our colleagues will help them to do so by becoming increasingly sensitive to the emotional processes that underlie healthy professional development. For all who read this book, we offer our wish that personally beneficial insights will result about the nature of personal development while pursing optimal career attainment in a highly demanding profession.

Contents

I

DEVELOPMENTAL STAGES IN THE PHYSICIAN'S CAREER

1

Pre-Medical and Medical School Training

Why would anyone seek involvement in a situation that requires giving up $100,000 of earned income while paying another $50,000 to an educational institution in order to work eighty hours a week for the next eight years under highly stressful conditions? A thoughtful person would question the motivation and wisdom of such an individual. Ruling out insanity as an explanation, one wonders what the ultimate payoff might be. Why would anyone pursue a course that requires so much sacrifice?

We speak, of course, of pre-med students, or, as they are less affectionately known by their peers, "grinds" or "science jocks." Willing to sacrifice much of the pleasure and freedom of their undergraduate years to attain a place in medical school, these students typically enroll in highly competitive and demanding science courses, and will not be satisfied with anything less than an "A". Then, to top it off, they willingly fly to distant cities at their own expense to undergo multiple interrogations by strangers who search for their defects.

Remarkably, nearly 40,000 medical school applicants in the United States submit each year to such ordeals. Moreover, of the 25,000 who do not win a place in medical school, most repeat the struggle the following year, or leave the country to participate in a similar ritual.

Clearly, considerable planning and personal commitment must be evident before one applies to medical school. But this was not always the case. During the early part of this century, medical schools had more available places than applicants. However, following the Flexner Report in the 1920s, many medical schools closed. Then during the 1930s, and 1940s, medicine embraced modern science, and thereafter basked in the prestigious flow of scientific knowledge and health-related technologies. As a medical career became a more glamorous career, the ratio of applicants to available places reversed dramatically. Increasing financial incentives and prestige enhanced by romanticized television dramas accelerated career appeal.

During application interviews, pre-med students characteristically express a desire to help people, yet maintain an involvement with science. Often noted is the inspiration received from physicians they have known. Rarely, though, do applicants mention parental pressures, prestige, or the economic rewards as a motivating factor. Application letters and interviews are remarkably similar in their expression of idealism.

Quantitative measures—grade point averages, especially in science courses, and scores on the Medical College Admission Test (MCAT)—are most typically used as the criteria for admitting applicants. These criteria are then used by the Association of American Medical Colleges to rank medical schools in prestige. Although considerable lip service is given to the value of attracting students from a broader base of interest and academic talent, tradition generally prevails.

So it is that nearly all physicians-to-be begin their training having been highly filtered to match a fairly uniform profile. The medical training system perpetuates itself by selecting applicants who come closest to matching its faculty—men rather than women, Anglo-Americans rather than minorities, and individuals who value "objectivity" and science rather than subjective feelings and humanistic interests.

While there may be little doubt that medical schools select some of the brightest, as measured by ability to recall detail and perform well on multiple-choice examinations, the question is whether they also attract those who will be the most interpersonally sensitive and well-balanced clinicians for the coming generations.

Having secured a place in medical school, students begin two years of basic science instruction followed by two years of clinical apprenticeship. The format for most of their basic science instruction, consisting primarily of lectures and laboratory work, is not dissimilar from their undergraduate experience, but the workload is much heavier and personal options considerably fewer.

Medical schools vary in the way they organize basic science materials. At some schools factual information is sequentially organized from microscopic (e.g., histology) to macroscopic (e.g., behavioral sciences), and from normality (physiology) to abnormality (pathology). At other schools, the organ system approach is utilized; information about kidneys or lungs, for example, is taught by various academic specialists as a unit. Sometimes information is presented without much logical sequence, depending on the availability and interest of the faculty. But whatever the approach, students spend most of their time in lecture halls passively listening, taking notes, and memorizing what will be needed for the next examination, which usually are of the multiple-choice format. In this regard, there is little diversity and no let up of pressure.

Entering students typically apply themselves energetically to mastering the materials, since they feel an awesome sense of obligation to future patients who may die because of their ignorance. Being serious-minded and dedicated is the norm in all of their endeavors. Willingness to work hard and to defer gratification has characterized their behavior thus far, and they anticipate that more of the same will be needed if they are to become successful physicians.

Though in possession of an excellent academic record, many students feel overwhelmed by the amount of material to be learned and intimidated by their classmates, all of whom initially appear to be brilliant. Incessant worries about the next exam, rarely more than two weeks away, dominate their thoughts. Because so little positive feedback is given during these early years, students push themselves hard and ruminate over minor errors. Constantly reminded that there are more facts to be mastered and that they do not know enough keeps them up reading late at night and prevents them from relaxing even when involved in recreational activities. Rather than enjoying a movie, for example, they worry that they are falling behind while their classmates are hard at work.

In the tightly structured learning environment, students have fewer options than they did as undergraduates and this, together with the routine, makes them feel stifled. Rather than being excited by their studies, some students find that the fun has gone out of learning, or that their minds have become stale. The "lockstepped forced-march routine" from lecture hall to lecture hall, from morning to late afternoon, five days a week, stifles independence, creativity, and enthusiasm. These young adults naturally have urges for youthful spontaneity and individuality. But few opportunities exist for expressing them.

In response to this learning environment, some students develop a mechanical method of rote learning, an approach that presumably carries over to patient care. Others become strident and rebellious, flaunting their individuality whenever possible. Most simply "go with the flow," dedicating themselves almost exclusively to their studies while neglecting other aspects of their lives.

Periodically, liberally oriented faculty members lobby for institutional changes that foster more individualized, creative thinking. But innovations, if adopted at all, rarely survive long. For example, when grades are eliminated in favor of a pass/fail evaluation system, national board scores typically drop, followed by faculty concern expressed in variations of the "I told you so" theme. The traditional grading system is then reestablished and the proper medical school ranking, as measured by student national board scores, is preserved. Homeostasis prevails.

A dramatic shift occurs near the beginning of the third year when the daily setting is changed from lecture hall and laboratory to the hospital floors. For most students this period stands out as the most critical period of their medical school training, one with the least certain outcome. Clerkships during the third year (medicine, surgery, pediatrics, ob/gyn, and psychiatry) and, to a lesser extent, the advanced clerkships of the fourth year are the heart of medical school training.

It is a rare student who feels any confidence before beginning these clerkships, and these feelings are heightened by hospital staff who ask, "haven't you learned that yet?" Yet just a few months earlier, others were saying, "Oh, don't worry, you will get that soon."

Patients are not hypothetical any more, not numbers in an equation; they are real people, sick people who are dependent on them; and this fact heightens anxieties. There is vast room for self-doubt as clinical students face up to their relative ignorance and wonder, "If I had only read that extra chapter, would I have learned something that would have prepared me better for this situation, or spared my patient some pain?" Worse yet is the concern, "Will my ignorance end up killing someone?" It is hard to believe, as students are told, that interns and residents will make sure this won't happen.

During the third and fourth years different learning skills are now required as a clinical "clerk." Gone are the days when one could do well simply by studying textbooks and lecture notes. No longer does the treatment of endocarditis, for example, or the most effective way to start an I.V. with a child, come recipe-style from a book. Nor is new material delivered in a sequential or predictable manner. A hospitalized patient who gives a clear, concise, and orderly history is as rare as a patient with leprosy. Students must organize and integrate important information not only from seriously ill, occasionally hostile patients who have already been interviewed two or three times by residents, interns, or others, but also from a variety of others—ward clerks, X-ray technicians, attending physicians, house staff, and sometimes the patients' relatives. Gathering and processing information this way can be bewildering, especially when the information leads to contradictory conclusions.

If not already realized, it now becomes overwhelmingly clear that not everything read or heard can be retained. So students must develop creative techniques to gather and retain needed information, a highly challenging task. Books, notes, and other aids are kept constantly at hand.

Completing one's work is also more logistically difficult. While trying to write up a case, a student may need to search for a lost X-ray or drop everything, for example, when ordered by the intern to draw an arterial blood gas. A scolding resident may ventilate about obstructing his light during a biopsy. While trying to meet these demands, fragments of conversation drift in from the hallway about fatal flaws to be avoided or other pearls of clinical wisdom. Trying to assimilate all this while meeting patient needs, receiving directions, being quizzed by instructors, and fitting in with the ward milieu creates a confusing matrix of demands that can be bewildering.

During the clinical years there is a rapidly shifting and confusing succession of quasi-roles: apprentice, lackey, student, patient advocate, doctor, klutz, clerk, the envied, the despised, and always the novice posing as expert. Because clinical students rotate to new assignments, the clerkship setting changes nearly every month, forcing them to cope not only with new logistical arrangements, but also with new patients, new team members, new procedures, new schedules, and new protocols. Allied health professionals that students never knew existed now demand information or issue orders.

Since so much of the learning during this time occurs in hospital settings, clinical corridors and organizational idiosyncrasies must be quickly mastered. As such, students often feel like a traveler in a foreign country. How late is the cafeteria open? Where are the chest films kept after 5:00? What is the phone number of the patient escort service? Where can my patient's family wait while I do the physical exam? How was I supposed to know that they don't do endoscopy on Friday?

Emotional management of these uncertainties is also complicated by major changes in personal lifestyle. During the basic science years students could at least count on sleeping at night in their own beds and, except for exam time, grabbing a bite to eat, getting some exercise, or visiting briefly with friends after classes. Now, their time is dictated by needs of patients, interns, or residents. Sleep is a luxury, and eating more of a fuel stop than a pleasure. Making concrete plans with the important people in one's life is a rarity. Also lost is the comfort that once came from the camaraderie and predictability of a hundred or so classmates all trooping together from one place to another, commenting on this or that ordeal. Instead, students are "shot-gunned" into forty separate clinical services or more, greatly increasing their sense of isolation and loneliness.

Underlying all this is the most chilling uncertainty of all: "Will I make the cut? After all the hard work and sacrifice, do I have what it takes to be a doctor? Will I really mess up and damage a patient? Will others realize how dangerously ill-equipped I feel? Can they sense my self-doubts? Will patients discover that I am not really a doctor, only a student masquerading as one—a fraud, an impostor who doesn't belong in a white coat?"

The one certainty of the clinical years is that "the real thing" is being experienced, a time to learn whether one has what it takes to be a physician. No amount of academic training can prepare them for such a time, for it challenges the sum of one's total life experience.

In this chapter six selections are presented to provide a more intimate glimpse of what life is like during the pre-med and medical school years. All but one were specially written for this book.

First, an introspective account of the pre-med experience is offered by Karen Axelsson in her article, "Pre-Med: A Personal Perspective." Since the author did not decide to become a pre-med student until age 25 (six or seven years older than most of her classmates), her perspective is most interesting and insightful. Having always despised pre-meds, Axelsson imagined them as "ruthless and competitive to the core." She was surprised, however, to find them different than imagined, although their motivations and ambitions remained a mystery to her. Colorfully portrayed are the anxieties, the hard work, the falling behind, then catching up, marking small triumphs and failures along the way, vacillating between hope and confidence and despair and dejection, but continuing to plug along until, finally, she was accepted to medical school.

Axelsson's account conveys the relentless self-doubt and struggle typically experienced by pre-med students as they face an uncertain outcome. The inner dialogue about whether one has the native ability to become a physician continues on throughout medical school.

The second selection is a brief narrative that deals with the medical school application process. "How I Got into Harvard Med,

Almost," by Marc Ringel, is a personal account of a medical school application interview, one that will ring true for anyone who has applied to medical school, especially at an elitist institution. His terse denouement captures the highly significant, yet unpredictable nature of the "luck of the draw," despite years of toil and sacrifice. Underscored in this amusing account is the importance of saying the right thing at the right time to the right person.

The next selection, another brief essay by Marc Ringel, deals with the technical vocabulary that must be mastered in medical school. "Calling a Spade a Terrestrial Excavation Implement" is an incisive reminder of how the inner sanctum of medical knowledge (and ignorance) is guarded by the three-headed Gorgon of obfuscation, esoterica, and reconditeness. Nevertheless, a knowledge of these medical passwords is critical if one is to gain entrance to the exclusive territory of medicine.

Possessed with the approved medical argot, a trainee can become an insider. Although a clinician may get by on the hospital wards with cowboy boots and unorthodox hair style, one cannot survive long if not familiar with the technical vocabulary. The author's lingua in buccal mucosa (tongue-in-cheek) style brings this point home perfectly. So, Ringel advises, keep a good medical dictionary handy, and look up every unknown medical word that comes up.

"Studies in the Anatomy Laboratory: A Portrait of Individual and Collective Defense" by Peter Finkelstein is a unique, in-depth study of the social and intrapsychic reactions of first-year medical students who dissect a human body. For ten hours a week during almost an entire year, students have the unusual experience of systematically dismantling another human body. The social and psychological dimensions of this experience are probed by Finkelstein, who devoted years to observing and interviewing those who undergo this otherwise forbidden activity. The author skillfully helps us see how this experience affects the psyche of a budding physician. Because the usual psychological defenses, such as avoidance and denial, cannot be utilized if one is to learn and pass exams, how do students cope? This and related questions are examined in this important analysis. Where else other than a morticians' school will a twenty-two year old be faced with the task of voluntarily cutting into and disemboweling a human body?

John McKinnon's article, "Sorcerer's Apprentice: Memoirs of a Medical Student," is a well-written overview of the medical school experience. Colorfully portrayed is the transition from the abstract knowledge gained in the first two years to the tangible, hands-on experiences of the third and fourth years. His discussion of the clinical clerkship offers a particularly good explanation of how medical students learn to stop thinking of themselves as students, and become doctors. The struggle towards competency, tinged with defeat each time a patient dies, provides a palpable quality to this description of medical training.

McKinnon's article captures with freshness and poignancy the excitement and the sadness that characterize the emotional experience of a sensitive person going through medical school. While some might question whether four years of medical school can be accurately compressed into such a brief account, the reader of this eloquent article will not be shortchanged.

Another thoughtful article, sensitively written, is Daniel Bressler's "Notes from Overground." We have selected this essay because it so clearly conveys the basic idealism that, although disguised or "underground" in most students, survives in medical school. Writing of his experiences as a fourth-year student, Bressler marvels at the privileged exposure he has had "to the underbelly and the hidden thoughts of humanity." Although medical training may have many defects, idealism, though tempered by reality, can for some remain undiminished.

Amidst all the problems, Bressler says, it is easy to forget or grow numb to the remarkable opportunities that routinely come in medical school. "But for few other people in society," he notes, "are the raw ingredients of life spread out so plainly in their beauty and ugliness. And on few others is the capacity to participate helpfully in another person's life bestowed so generously."

The final selection in this chapter highlights a heretofore neglected topic, the experiences of American students at foreign medical schools. Strangely, almost nothing has been written about this topic, despite the fact that, in the United States, nearly one-fourth of all licensed physicians with permanent residency status are foreign medical graduates. Some of these physicians were born and raised outside of the United States, while others were American students who, because they were unable to gain acceptance into U.S. medical schools, left the country to study in foreign lands.

"Gringo-boy Comes Home to Practice Medicine," by Robert Coombs, is a grim account of two American students who trained at a medical school in Latin America. Those who undergo such experiences must be highly determined, adaptable, and psychologically strong if they are to survive.

The plight of the foreign-trained physician is different in many respects from that of their American-trained counterparts. They must move to a foreign country, learn a new language, adapt to strange customs, and perhaps experience prejudice and discrimination. Moreover, the quality of training by comparison with American schools may not be up to standard.

Having endured all of this, these graduates must pass qualifying exams before they can continue their training in the United States and if successful, complete an extra year of clinical training called a "fifth pathway" year. These are the lucky ones. After investing enormous personal resources in their foreign training, some are not allowed to practice in their homeland.

The so-called "doctor glut" has focused considerable attention on foreign medical schools and reduced the number of opportunities to practice in America. News accounts, editorials, and even cartoons have highlighted the dilemma and caught the attention of the American public. Should there be greater or fewer restrictions on doctors entering the United States? The answer is not simple, especially when considering humanistic complexities of those who have endured years of stressful experiences and invested enormous resources in their foreign training.

Pre-Med: A Personal Perspective

Karen Axelsson

I came late in life to the desire for doctorhood. At 25, when I returned to school to fulfill pre-med requirements, I felt light-years removed from my fellow med school aspirants. In college, I had always despised pre-meds, imagining them ruthless and competitive to the core. Returning to take pre-med courses, I felt like someone who had stumbled into an enemy camp, only to find it manned by children. The fresh faces around me from NY and LA and Cincinnati were only 18 or 19. They seemed naive and confident, already at this tender age planning careers in medical research to be conducted at the top institutions in America. In contrast, I had spent years girding up to announce my desire to be a doctor—years of working in low-paying human service jobs, years of questioning whether I was wise enough and sensitive enough to be a helper, years of imagining that only people more intelligent and accomplished than I would be considered for admission to medical school. It was a point of existential reckoning that sent me back to do pre-med, knowing that not to try would be a demoralizing admission of defeat, yet unable to imagine my quest would ever be successful. Thus it was not surprising that the easy self-confidence and ambition of my fellow students was mysterious to me. What motivated them, I wondered, and what did they dream of as they thought of their future careers? Did they worry at all as I had at their age about whether they would be good enough helpers to people who had sustained tragedy? Would they grow into their roles as physicians naturally and gracefully, or would the sadness and strain of medicine be too much for them to accomodate right out of college? I pondered these questions, and decided there were no generalized answers. I met lovely and sincere students, as well as some who mainly seemed to contemplate the glories of radiology, making 200 G's a year, and having 6 weeks of paid vacation. Although their youth and innocence quickly demolished my monstrous images of them, my classmates remained mysterious to me, and I to them. Consequently, I concentrated on my own efforts in school and left them alone.

Pre-med was a combination of nightmare and triumph. Always in the background was the anxiety that all this was only to apply, with no guarantees of acceptance. The possibility of wasting two years on a quest that would ultimately prove futile seemed an apocalyptic nightmare to me. Since my eventual selection from among tens of thousands of applicants seemed so remote, I focused on shorter-term goals, doing the best I could in every class. I went at my studies with unprecedented vengeance. Whenever my motivation or energy started to founder, I imagined not getting into school and how I would feel if I had to attribute this to my own mediocre effort. Needless to say, the distractions of the moment just never seemed worth it.

It is hard for those already initiated to realize just how utterly fantastic the reality portrayed in science is to the newcomer. I approached my first biology class with all the wonderment and disbelief of a native Papuan watching an airplane fly overhead. My professor was a well-meaning man who totally lacked the capacity to organize his lectures; thus, every day I was taken on a careening exploration of scientific fact which ranged from DNA repair mechanisms in yeast to the Hardy–Weinberg equation of population genetics. Having no science background, everything he related seemed improbable to me and I was completely unable to gauge the accuracy of my comprehension. Sitting in a dark lecture hall with electron micrographs flashing before me, I lost track of every lecture several minutes into it, and sat scribbling notes furiously, leaving large gaps and dotting every line with question marks. Was everyone so confused? My young classmates seemed remarkably unperturbed by all of this. Did this presage doom for my dreamed-of career? Somehow, despite this daily anxiety, I was eventually able to grasp the internal logic of the material, helped immensely by outside reading and my aggressive pursuit of teaching assistants. I was not, however, able to master my primitive doubts that any of these submicroscopic biological processes occurred in the real world.

My worst trial by fire came the next quarter in that infamous pre-med course, organic chemistry. Even buying the text was intimidating. In an era when textbook authors and publishers seemed to strive for accessibility, the book's cover was a solid and sober dark blue, and its weight engendered jokes that it could double as a weapon of self-defense. At least in this class, I knew I was not alone in my fear and confusion. The two hundred and fifty odd freshmen and I were all united in our apprehension as the professor sailed blithely into his initial lecture on this terrifying and mysteriously important subject. Years of familiarity with the area had obscured his sense of how to make this material intelligible to neophytes, and it was not until months later that I finally grasped what all this fuss over carbon was about. During the first mid-term, the tension in the lecture hall was palpable. There was not enough time to finish the examination, and when I got my test back several days later, I found I had gotten a 77—a solid C. I was undone. The small buds of confidence which had grown the previous quarter abruptly vanished, and utter failure and humiliation loomed on the horizon. I was obsessed over the implications of this mediocre performance for the next week, breaking into tears every time I envisioned my dream slipping away. Finally, I realized that I could not afford to think about it any longer. Instead, I concentrated single-mindedly on mastering organic chemistry, studiously avoiding all thought of the future. Page by page, problem by problem, I forged ahead, cornering the head TA for hours each week to review problems and manipulate plastic hydrocarbon models with me.

Working so hard made it difficult for my constantly lurking anxiety to really get a grip, and the success which resulted from this intensive labor eventually made me confident of my ability to master the pre-med curriculum. Unfortunately, it made me no more confident of getting a spot in medical school. In my imagination, I competed with 1,000's of 4.0 pre-meds, and having a good GPA just seemed to put me in the middle of the pack, with no particular advantage. I banked most of my slim hopes for distinction on being able to impress medical schools with my greater than average maturity and life experience. I knew that an essay addressing why one wanted to be a doctor was a part of every standard medical school application. I hoped, in this section, to elaborate on the personal characteristics that I really did feel would make me a good doctor, and to turn things that might be perceived negatively into positive selling points. Knowing that this would be my only opportunity to distinguish myself, I was aghast to find, upon picking up the application form, that I had only one side of a piece of paper on which to accomplish this. `

Writing the "good enough" essay proved to be a 3-month ordeal. It was by far the most difficult and discouraging part of the pre-med experience for me. It brought me face to face with all the internal self-doubts and insecurities I could ignore while studying fiendishly, but which leapt up to mock me as I tried to write an honest statement of how I had come to this point. Writing the essay also brought the whole pursuit a step closer to reality, and since my vivid imaginings had thus far only included rejection, it was an uncomfortable reality to contemplate. Confronted with the necessity of revealing my deepest dreams to anonymous admissions panels across the country, I imagined the worst—a nation-wide network either amused or irritated at my audacity in applying. Why, I had not even received grades at my undergraduate college, and now I thought I could just waltz right into medical school!

Finally, in late August, after numerous drafts and alternating fits of despondency, I completed the applications. Pleased with my essay but full of misgiving about all the things I had not been able to list as accomplishments, I submitted them to the local post office. They were destined for 26 medical schools. I would have applied to many more, but I had exhausted the list of those located anywhere that I thought I could bear living for four years.

That fall, an undergraduate teaching assistant who was also applying to medical school directed my vertebrate biology lab. Full of success from his four years at this prestigious private institution, he had already had two medical school inteviews and had requests for several more. With burgeoning self-importance, he related the newest application developments to our class each week. After finding out that I was also applying for next year, he questioned me weekly, "Had I heard anything yet?" "No," I kept replying, cursing him inwardly for this quiet torture. After 6 weeks or so, he finally stopped, seemingly bored or embarrassed by my apparent failure.

Soon afterward, my first invitation to interview came from the Ivy League. I will remember forever that moment of staring at the monographed red letterhead and reading the cordial invitation to come and speak about a place in next year's medical school class. A wild surge of awe and relief spread through me as I realized that someone out there on that great anonymous admissions panel had actually seen my application, had in fact singled it out from among thousands of applications. Maybe it did not matter that I had floundered for years in choosing a profession, that I hadn't grown up winning science fairs or worked in any Nobel laureate's lab, that I'd only returned to school last year feeling like an overgrown, hulking child to discover what a cell was and to perform hackneyed chemistry experiments. Maybe they would let me in anyway. As instructed in the letter, I called up the school to arrange for an interview. While the phone rang, I cleared my throat, wanting desperately to sound calm and poised, as if arranging for a medical school interview was an everyday event for me. Fortunately, the person who answered the phone was less anxious than I, and carried most of the conversation while smoothly arranging an appointment for me. Hanging up, I was suddenly fascinated with an actuarial analysis of my situation. I pulled out my pre-med bible, the catalogue of medical schools, and looked up what percentage of applicants were interviewed at this Ivy League medical college. Then I calculated what percentage of interviewed applicants were accepted. Statistically, my chances were 45%. Not bad, I thought.

After I had received several more of these delightful missives, reality began to hit. Following this triumphant period of recognition, I was actually going to have to sit down with faculty from the country's foremost colleges and discuss my future career in medicine. My imaginary competition changed from the young pre-med coterie whom I had handily defeated, to that eminently intelligent and accomplished cadre that had so intimidated me as an under-graduate. I had no publications or accomplishments or great feats of leadership to speak of. What would I talk about? My interviewers would surely see through me, reading the insecurity I knew would be written all over my face. This was not what they looked for in future doctors. Friends gently pointed out to me that my expecta-tions of myself might be just a tad high. Interviewers would probably not expect a doctoral dissertation or a candidate with absolutely no interview anxiety. What did they expect of me then? I moaned. I knew it would be something I did not have.

Over the next month, I did psychological double-time, rework-ing my image of myself to include "future MD," and re-molding the concept of "future MD" to include me. Gradually, I began to feel that it would not represent a gross miscalculation on someone's part if I were eventually picked to become a doctor. By the time I finally got to my interviews, I had to giggle inwardly at the outlandishness of my initial apprehensions. There was indeed one interviewer who caricatured my fears perfectly, starting off our talk by asking me to account for my mid-life career change, and later snidely suggesting that I would probably begin to dream of being a concert pianist after finishing my medical degree. The numerous other interviews I had were delightful and illuminating. I met people I hadn't expected to find in medicine—wise and humane, from diverse backgrounds, concerned about the problems facing the profession today—in short, a far cry from the established caucasian brotherhood I'd imagined. They seemed respectful and eager to know about me, and I began to feel comfortable in relating how I'd come to this point, my values in medicine, and my dreams for the future.

By the time I'd finished the interviews, I knew my pre-med journey was nearing its end. I felt like a very different person from when I'd started. I'd grown a lot through this experience and now had a whole new life ahead of me. I knew my new challenges and fears and acts of courage would take place while becoming a doctor.

How I Got into Harvard Med, Almost

Marc Ringel

When I applied to medical school there were about half as many freshman class slots for us baby boomers as there are now. Competition was further intensified by the availability of medical student deferments for the Vietnam draft. Consequently, I applied to 18 medical schools, a modest number in those days. Among them was Harvard.

I didn't like Harvard from the first. It was the only school that did not send me the catalogue I requested, explaining it was available at most college libraries. Then there was the application—they wanted a high-school transcript and writing sample. Unlike other applications, which were to be printed or typed, Harvard's was to be typed, period.

Apparently, I got over the first hurdle well enough to qualify for an interview. They sent a man by my college campus as a side trip to his main job of recruiting minority students.

We met at the information desk of the student union. I showed up in a funky pair of jeans, sandals, shirt, tie and sports jacket. I was sporting a scraggly goatee and a curly mop of hair.

When I arrived there was a man standing at the desk facing away from me. I spoke the name of my inquisitor-to-be. He turned and responded, smiling. He was wearing funky jeans, sandals, jacket and tie, scraggly goatee, and long curly hair.

We sat for 2 or 3 hours drinking coffee at a booth in the union discussing enthusiastically politics, science, and philosophy. I extemporaneously developed that afternoon the song and dance that was to serve me well at most of my future medical school interviews. I found that nearly every question I was asked by my various interviewers was a variation of "Why do you want to be a doctor?"

I answered that question well enough in the eyes of my mirror image to be asked back for a second round of interviews. By the time Harvard told me they wanted me to come to Boston, I had already been accepted at several schools. I wasn't about to drop everything and travel thousands of miles just so they could look at me again, not even for Harvard. So I asked if they might find somebody locally who could interview me.

They chose an alumnus, the Chief of Pathology of a large Chicago hospital. I was a bus driver for the Chicago Transit Authority at the time so I wore a regulation moustache (not past the corners of my mouth) and matching haircut. I even wore shoes and wash slacks to go with my jacket and tie. Given the formality of my interviewer and of the institution in which he worked, it was a fortunate choice. But no clothes or shoes, not even new, well-polished, all-leather, black Florsheim wing tips with cleats could have kept me from stepping off a cliff that day.

It started innocently enough. We were strolling down one of the byways of the big why-do-you-want-to-be-a-doctor question. I had been explaining why I wanted to be a psychiatrist. My interviewer asked wouldn't psychology have been a better major than philosophy, given my career goals? I told him I didn't like the brand of psychology taught at my university. It was too behaviorist, I explained, even Skinnerian. I elaborated on the evils of Skinner's reductionist views of the human psyche, not really expecting this pathologist to follow.

He did. "B. F. Skinner," he said. "Genius. My room mate at Harvard."

That fall I enrolled at the School of Medicine of the University of Illinois.

Calling a Spade
a Terrestrial Excavation Implement

Marc Ringel

A new medical journal, among the several dozen free ones I receive every month, purports to tell us physicians how to market our practices. One of their recommendations to keep us looking marketably up to date is to have new-appearing medical books displayed in our offices. I'm glad to say that I do. I even look at those books now and then.

One book which is not up to date is my *Steadman's Medical Dictionary*. I bought it in 1970, when I started medical school. Though I hardly use it now, it was the most important book I owned as a medical student.

Medical language is a world unto itself. Its long words and the acronyms that sometimes stand in their stead may encode whole universes of important meaning in a terse shorthand. T.E.N.S., I.T.P., and A.I.D.S. say a lot to a fluent speaker. This form of communication is also capable of producing remarkably long, obfuscating ways of saying simple things. An idiopathic erythematous exanthem of the axilla is merely a red rash of the armpit, cause unknown. Epistaxis secondary to digital trauma is a bloody nose from picking it.

Medical language, a clumsy combination of Latin and Greek roots, prefixes, and suffixes mingled with archaic English and seasoned with German and French, probably serves more to inhibit good communication between physicians and the lay public than any other single factor. Have you ever noticed how doctors interviewed on talk and news shows "visualize" rather than "see," talk about "tympanic membranes" rather than "ear drums," feel "induration" rather than a "lump," probe the "superior aspect of the glabella" rather than the "upper surface of the forehead" where they may encounter a "hematoma" rather than a "bruise"? And these people are trying to communicate!

Talking, thinking, and writing like that becomes a habit. Whether you like it or not, to be a physician, you have to be able to do it. Even if you try to remember to call an arm an "arm," you have to know what your colleagues mean when they talk about an "upper extremity."

Which brings me to the point of the column. Buy a medical dictionary as soon as you're accepted to medical school—*Steadman's, Dorland's,* or *Taber's*—it doesn't really matter. Look up every medical word you encounter that you don't know or even feel a bit hazy about. If you don't understand the language, you cannot learn anything else. Besides, it does allow you to sound pretty darned smart even when all of medical science is in the dark about the subject at hand. When you tell your prospective partner, whom you just met in a bar, that you diagnosed a child with FLK syndrome (s)he will probably be impressed. You may blow your plans for the rest of the evening though if you translate FLK. It means, "funny looking kid," a *bona fide* diagnosis.

Studies in the Anatomy Laboratory: A Portrait of Individual and Collective Defense

Peter Finkelstein

Within a week of starting medical school most students find themselves in a large, antiseptic laboratory, dissecting a preserved human body. The prevailing belief is that the laboratory experience is emotionally routine or, in the language of clinical medicine, "unremarkable." This may be seen most simply in the design of the typical anatomy course. But detailed observation of over 300 students in this four-year study shows that despite the professional detachment that the school expects of them, students' responses to the gross anatomy dissection lab are neither routine nor unremarkable.

Students' responses to this new experience, as shown publicly by their behavior in lab and privately by their dreams and subjective reports, were the subject of a four-year study of medical students that I conducted in the anatomy laboratory of a medical school at a private university in the western United States. Three hundred forty students took part, roughly 85 from each class. From them I gathered daily accounts of dreams and comments about their subjective experiences. Questionnaire data were obtained from a single random sample of 35 students, in order to answer specific questions and to involve students who did not volunteer information. Additional data were drawn from more than 200 hours of lab observation, and 60 hours of observation of faculty at their weekly planning meetings.

Results of the study show that in the anatomy lab many students do encounter a pointed challenge to their existing adaptive strategies. They both exhibit their response publicly in their talk and humor in the lab, and conceal aspects of their subjective responses from their teachers and colleges. These signs and symptoms have much to tell about the deeper experience of medical training, as the anatomy lab is but the first of student-doctors' many encounters with illness and death. Such encounters provide a series of instructions in "the clinical attitude," the attitude it is hoped students will master in order to behave intelligently and gracefully in the face of calamity. These encounters are an instruction in the management of emotion in extreme circumstances.

THE ANATOMY COURSE

The Curriculum

From the faculty's point of view the purpose of the first-year laboratory course in gross anatomy is to equip students with a working knowledge of body structure in considerable detail. This task is made difficult by the enormous amount of material and the difficulty in precisely determining the core knowledge for a first-year student of the subject.

It has been estimated that before qualifying as a doctor, a medical student must master 10,000 new terms; three-quarters of these terms arise in the study of gross anatomy (Christensen and Telford). A recent American edition of *Gray's Anatomy* contained 1,257 pages with 780 illustrations, and while students are not expected to master each page of such a volume, they are expected to commit major portions of it to memory, and to gain familiarity with every major anatomic area. Towards that end, the course under study contained 180 hours of classwork in less than six months. Three-quarters of this time is spent in the dissection laboratory.

The group's task during these lab sessions was to find specific body structures detailed in lecture and manual, free them physically from surrounding fat and extraneous tissue, demonstrate the structures, and memorize them, including their relation to adjacent anatomic features. At times the faculty used previously dissected bodies or body-parts in order to demonstrate critical structures, but the guiding expectation was that students learn the material through the dissection of their assigned cadaver.

One or two hours of lecture preceding each lab session prepared the students for dissection. The year's lecture schedule contained several hours of clinically related talks—for example, lectures on facial injury or lumbar disc disease—but most lectures were taken up with the basic science of anatomy. To supplement these lectures, and to bridge the gap from book anatomy to dissection in lab, smaller and less formal talks were given in the lab proper, sometimes to as few as eight or ten students.

In talking about the anatomy lab, students inevitably empha- sized the large number of facts they had to master; they learned early that academic quarters move quickly and that a great deal is covered between late September and the week before Christmas. Students described medical school science courses as conceptually easier than undergraduate science courses, but said they were far more demanding in quantity and often a good deal less rewarding for just this reason. First-year students frequently felt deluged and inade- quate in the face of their several courses, hard exams, and vivid con- cern that what they didn't know might maim some future patient.

The Setting

The Anatomy lab suite at the university where I conducted the study was composed of three large, high-ceilinged, rectangular rooms, each large enough to hold six to eight dissection tables. The rooms were white-walled and well-lit from above; shiny aluminum dissec- tion tables rested in rows on dark linoleum floors. Each room had a large blackboard and at least one sink where students washed instruments and rinsed anatomic specimens. Equipment used in the course—pumps, large standing lights, electric saws, chisels, drills, and the like—stood in the corners of the large rooms. Each room had its own X-ray view boxes which were covered with X-rays pertinent to the week's dissection. Often there was a weekly quiz question attached to one of the X-rays.

Students came into the lab for their first session within a few days of the start of classes. When they entered, prepared by a short introductory lecture, their first task was to ready the cadaver for dissection. Resting upon each of the twenty-odd aluminum tables was a black plastic body bag made of heavy vinyl and zipped shut. Inside the plastic bag, the cadaver was wrapped in cheesecloth saturated with formaldehyde. This moist medium is critical for the preservation of the body over the several months of dissection. The maintenance of this moisture and the proper wrapping of the body at the close of every dissection period comprised the student's most basic responsibility. In this particular lab, as in many anatomy labs, the face and limbs were covered by additional cheesecloth wraps until students reached that area of the dissection.

The appearance of the body changed steadily during the several months of dissection. As the internal cavities were opened up, organs had to be removed, both so that they could be studied, and so that access to other, deeper organs could be achieved. In order, for example, to visualize the bottom of the chest cavity, lungs and heart were freed from their surrounding structures and laid down beside the body while further dissection was in progress. At the close of each lab period students had to replace the contents of chest or abdomen and rewrap the body in damp cheesecloth. Often the wrapped body was wet further with tap water poured from a plastic watering can.

By the final weeks of most anatomy courses the body is typically in several pieces, with most of the internal structures removed to sit adjacent to the body on the rim of the table. At some schools the limbs are separated from the body. The head is typically removed from the neck, and the skull is further cut in at least two sections. At some schools the body is cut into halves or even quarters, to permit fuller visualization of internal structures. Fat and subcutaneous tissue is removed at each stage of the dissection, so that the mass of the body is gradually reduced from the start of the course to its conclusion. By the last week of the course the body has been emptied of most of its vital structures, leaving intact only the "chassis" of exposed muscle and bone.

To aid students in learning specific anatomic areas, previously prepared dissections—prosections—were used for demonstration by faculty or were available upon request. These prosected parts, for example, limbs and heads, were stored in large aluminum bins labeled on the outside with masking tape, according to the body parts inside. A container might then be labeled "limbs," or "heads."

When lab was in progress, each table was surrounded by the customary group of four students, the working team unit. Students on the four-member teams informally divided up the functions necessary to proceed with lab. One student might be responsible for clarifying anatomic details of the region, another for finding the most helpful illustrations from the available atlases; a third student might perform the actual dissection with probe and scalpel. Often these roles were exchanged over time, but it was not uncommon to find students who mainly dissected and others who dissected rarely.

The general ambience in the working lab was one of cheerful collegiality and quick movement. There was much talk, much noise from instruments, procedures, drains, and saws. A stereo sound system played light jazz and soft rock music. Less often, a classical station played Bach or Beethoven. Students visited one another's tables to learn anatomy but also to socialize; although the work was long and often tedious, most students reported that they had a good time in the lab.

In lab, students rushed about, asked questions, borrowed suction pumps, and looked at the anatomy on adjacent cadavers. There was a great deal of talk. For the many students who felt that they learned best through dissection, long periods of careful handwork were required to best demonstrate critical structures. Much of the time this dissection work was going on, students were busy with their hands, probing and cutting, but free to pursue their own improvised conversation or thought. Only when they found the searched-for structure, for example, an artery or nerve, did they have to pay careful attention and commit detail to memory. Between discoveries students had plenty of time to talk casually or even horse around while the manual work proceeded.

It is generally accepted that Gross Anatomy is the central course of the first year of medical school, and that it forms the basis for later study in pathology, physical exam, radiology, and the various subspecialties of surgery. It is, furthermore, often the students' favorite course, and is designated by many students as the course that makes them feel most like physicians-to-be.

The explicit course of anatomy includes the physical work of dissection and the enormous amount of material that the student must master. These are the concrete elements of the course. But if one includes the unspoken task of adapting to these vivid reminders of death and aging, it becomes a far more complex course to conceive of—for in parallel with these concrete elements, students must quietly learn to handle their responses to the dead body and what it represents to them.

The Implicit Course

Working in conjunction with the concrete details of the lab setting, unspoken social norms help define the rules and boundaries of acceptable behavior. They spell out for the student what the expectations are for behavior within the lab, what should be noticed and what should be ignored or forgotten.

The most encompassing norm within the anatomy lab is the complex requirement for professional conduct. Students are expected to "act like a doctor," even on the third day of medical school. They are expected to place their acquisition of knowledge above all other priorities, to treat the cadaver, their first patient, with respect, and to deal with any emotional responses they may have to the situation in private. Displays of true anxiety or sorrow are tacitly discouraged, but shows of frustration or disappointment about progress in mastering the cognitive material are acceptable—and common.

Often, students were shown sights or asked to carry out procedures that were startling or even shocking to them. They were seldom prepared for these experiences, for it was assumed that their responses will be negligible.

Since students were uniformly reluctant to comment to instructors on the disturbing nature of the material, dramatic events were only reviewed in private conversations. The information loop from students back to faculty was thus diverted by social norms and imagined expectations. As such, this pattern perpetuated a partial misunderstanding about the nature of students' experience.

A color-slide presentation about facial injuries was one startling event; a film showing the exposed nerves in the arm of an anesthetized woman whose arm had just been amputated, was another. A third example, commented upon by many students, was the use of a stillborn child's body to demonstrate anatomic features not found in adult bodies. Several students dreamt about the moment when the child's body was hoisted up onto their own cadaver unexpectedly by an enthusiastic instructor. A final example was the procedure where the top of the intact skull was sawed through horizontally and the upper portion of the brain removed with one cut of a large flat knife. In each of these situations the clear expectation was that the students would master the information at hand, then go about their business as before.

At weekly planning meetings, faculty discussions of the course were limited to the logistics of teaching and demonstration; the overriding concern for the teaching faculty was to design an approach to the anatomic region under study which would yield the best learning experience for students. Often the faculty deliberated between two alternative approaches, each showing one aspect of the anatomy more clearly than another; there was a sustained interest in improving the course from quarter to quarter and from year to year. The emotional reactions of students to the course, since the faculty assumed them to be negligible, received no attention during staff meetings. When the faculty found the dissection of the perineum and genitals proceeding at too slow a pace they explained it in terms of the difficulty of the anatomic planes.

This school was far from unique in this respect. Most medical schools around the country overlook the emotional response of students, beginning even *before* they enter medical school. It is common practice at many schools to escort the medical school applicant through the anatomy suite on the day he or she is on campus for the admissions interview. One applicant told me of being led into the anatomy suite of an old elite Eastern medical school shortly before fall term finals, only to find two students rolling a head across the floor. Another applicant described how he was whisked into the anatomy suite by an enthusiastic guide who marched his charges, without warning, through rows of bodies to the far side of the lab, where he leapt energetically onto the last counter to exclaim over the view of the bay.

The explicit course in Gross Anatomy is the learning of anatomic structure through lecture, audiovisual aid, and dissection lab. This curriculum receives a great deal of attention from the faculty, quite understandably; to many of them this explicit curriculum represents the entire course. But another course exists, implicit in the experiences of students, and it, too, may be characterized.

The message for the first-year student is implicit but it comes consistently from many directions: study hard and learn a lot; learn to be objective; there is little place in the practice of medicine for the subjective response. Such norms govern the outward display of students' emotions, and in doing so, help define the process of coming to terms with that which is disturbing. But such norms can regulate only certain sectors of behavior. Eventually, anxiety, depression, or some translated form of coping appear elsewhere, outside the jurisdiction of such unspoken rules. It is in this fashion that the anatomy lab shapes not only knowledge, but also values, behavior, and even emotional responsiveness, which the student later brings to medical work.

STUDENT RESPONSES TO THE ANATOMY COURSE

Though a variety of constraints upon students' responses were outlined in the preceding sections, students do, willy nilly, learn their anatomy and fashion some response to the emotional issues at hand. Some responses are individual and some are collective, fashioned by the group, or encouraged by the subculture. Talk, nonverbal behavior in the lab, and humor are each public and collective to varying extents, and they may reveal aspects of students' preoccupations that are not generally acknowledged.

Language and Talk in the Laboratory

Since the acquisition of a new language is a central task in students' first two years of medical training, and since professional language so clearly mediates between actor and environment, language is uniquely suited to play a defensive role with respect to the students' new experience. The following excerpt is from the basic laboratory manual used in the course:

> Prior to dissection of muscles, due consideration must be given to the superficially positioned mammary gland. The thoracic wall is covered anteriorly by muscles which belong to the upper limb. These muscles (pectoralis major and minor; subclavius) must be dissected and reflected before the intercostal spaces and their contents can be approached. Subsequently, the anterior thoracic wall will be removed to provide access to the thoracic cavity. (Grant's Dissector, 8th Edition, Williams and Wilkins, 1978)

This paragraph outlines the approach to the dissection of the breast and the chest wall. It exemplifies the formal language of anatomic description; as such, it carries forward the norms of scientific objectivity and masculine reserve; it is a precise language which does not allow for students' subjectivity as it fulfills its technical purpose. Understandably, the student imitates this way of talking and learns to use it freely. It is a useful style of talk for it permits accurate communication of anatomic information. Moreover, it grants to the user that sense of mastery so critical to the novice in medicine. In this manner of talk, one dissects, reflects, and exposes; one does not cut, peel, or poke. One dissects anatomic material; one does not look backward to the person once invested in this body.

If the formal language of anatomy is appealing for the sense of control it affords, the informal language of the laboratory offers a mastery more colorful and full of humorous possibility:

> We seem to do more hacking when the positive ions are in the air, donch'ya think?

The above remark and many like it represent a different talk, improvised and often humorous, which goes on interspersed with the formal. Students talk about "hacking", "whacking", and "muti-lating." It is a rough talk, full of what one student referred to as "the obvious bravado," and is often intermingled with humor. This talk, too, is protective, but it differs from the formal talk of the lab both in poking fun at the process and in indirectly acknowledging a more aggressive aspect to students' own participation.

The language of medicine neutralizes experience and renders it more palatable. It is as if the experiences of doctoring are predigested by this discourse, the fresh impact already filtered by a latinate and formal system of references. Language, as Lifton points out, is a prime conveyor of psychic numbing. This is evident in clinical medicine where the coronary artery bypass graft operation is referred to as a "Cabbage (CABG)," and the removal of kidneys from young people killed in motor vehicle accidents referred to as the "harvesting" of kidneys. Such clinical talk seems similar to much of that in the anatomy lab: the impact of direct experience is diminished by the interpolation of language.

Behavior

If the words of the lab manual renamed the vast amount of cutting, pulling, scraping, poking, and the like which went on at dissection, these activities went on, nonetheless. And as they went on, one afternoon after another, some students began to elaborate upon their dissective duties: they added to or modified the tasks at hand. These extra behaviors often revealed a noteworthy attempt to dehumanize the cadaver.

During certain periods of the course, it was common to observe students using body parts to perform practical functions at the laboratory table. Portions of the brain, often the cerebellum, were used as scalpel-holders. Additional berths for the dissection knives were fashioned out of liver. Solid organs like the liver and the spleen were used as pillows for the head and the neck. The top of the skull, as well, was used to position other parts of the body.

> At one table I noted that four scalpels were sticking into the cadaver's back, marking off a small square area. At another table a single knife was sticking vertically out of a cadaver's back. The student quietly removed the scalpel from the back as he saw me approach.
> At another table, the last portion of the cadaver's penis was cut off transversely in a manner not accounted for by the direction

in the lab manual. Two of the women joked that this was revenge for the vulgar joke of their male tablemate.

This behavior may be understood as an attempt to tame the body. The use of the brain to hold dissection knives removes the awesome associations we have to the brain as seat of the intelligence, even the soul. The behavior domesticates the brain by turning it into a knife rack, like in the kitchen.

At one table students had transplanted several glands and rearranged the cadaver's anatomy with several procedures not outlined in the manual.

Such rearrangement of the anatomy as seen in this last example was quite rare, although the use of liver or brain to aid in the dissection, or the performance of small extra cuttings or stabbings, were not.

Late in the course, while dissecting the head, students began to quietly discuss the possibility of removing gold teeth from the cadavers.

I have no knowledge that this was actually done in the lab observed, though it is striking that it was seriously contemplated; it is common knowledge, though not commonly acknowledged, that removal of teeth does occur at some medical schools during some class years. The rationale usually offered is that such gold is no longer of use to the cadaver and is wasted in cremation. Underneath such pragmatism, is, perhaps, the more psychological rationale: I am owed something for being subjected to this yellow abdomen, aged genitals, and generally unpleasant experience. How else can we explain that conscientious and honest young people entertain—and sometimes do—what they would normally think to be well beyond their rights and privileges? This oddly rough behavior may be understood as an attempt to distance the experience by de-emphasizing the previous life of the cadaver. If the body is stripped of the rights and consideration given to the living, it is lowered both in status and in its capacity to arouse emotion.

Student Humor

Among the collective behaviors elaborated by students in the laboratory, none is so striking as the production of humor. It is students' laughter and high spirits that determine the ambience of the lab from day to day. The humor is very densely packed. For simple purposes of definition, let us say that humor is that which results in laughter, or is clearly intended to achieve that end. It may depend upon a sight gag or facial expression, but in the anatomy lab it is usually communicated in the talk which accompanies the work.

The following seven examples of humor were culled from hundreds noted during laboratory sessions.

> A red balloon with white lettering was tied to one of the dissection tables in the front room and rose upward filled with helium. It said "Lively Arts Festival."

> Student, while holding up a white packaging string soaked in fluid: "What's this, a nerve?" He then tossed it into the abdominal cavity. "We'll throw it over there, and later when we find it we'll call it a nerve!"

This joke, which resulted in a round of laughter, seemed to derive its spark from the speaker's infectious high spirits, and from his concise reference to the huge task which lay before them. It suggested that anatomic reality might be rewritten with a toss of the wrist. The student who made this and many other winning jokes was also having disturbing lab-related dreams at night. The first dream in the following section, about the mother who had died and was wandering around lost and crying, was dreamt by this same student, within days of the above joking.

> Two students are talking in front of a prosected leg (one which has been dissected carefully by the staff to reveal several layers of well-defined anatomic structure). Student one, imitating a scholarly British accent and pretending to be part of a two-person surgical team: "This is disgusting. What a terrible job—gangrene I think. Should we operate? I think when it comes off with a pliers, that's the criteria I use." Second student: "Should we warm it first?"

This student, seeming to fashion his surgical team after Hawkeye and his buddy from "Mash," was also the student who admitted on the last day of the course to having been frightened in the lab at night and to ritually having to count bodies to "prepare for" a fantasied uprising. The high spirits of such horseplay serve well to quiet anxiety, in part by their invocation of an intrepid duo, armed with knowledge, privilege, and the spirit of adventure.

I approach two students working at the foot of a table and see one student pushing his scalpel into the cadaver's heel. Just as he pushes the scalpel into the heel again, the student turns to me and asks, "Want to see how I get the reflexes?" The sound of the scalpel penetrating the gritty connective tissue was faintly audible as he repeated the gesture. The two students laughed.

The presence or absence of "reflexes" on the cadaver was the focus for many jokes, most of them corny but, in context, somehow irresistible. This joke added a small pinch of violence to that standard formula.

Some students joked about considering dog and cat names for the cadavers. One table of four women talked about naming their cadaver for their former husbands' current wives.

Not all cadavers were named, but many were, as has been the tradition for generations. Although naming is sometimes explained as an attempt to humanize the cadaver, this seems unlikely since the assigned names are invariably ones of social distance, uncommon in the middle classes of this generation. Names like Ernest (for "dead-ernest"), Loretta, and Bertha abound. One seldom finds students naming a cadaver Robert or Ellen. Naming always emphasized the cadaver's origination somewhere else, geographically, socially, or ethnically.

In one telling example of naming, a practicing physician recalled that the cadaver he worked on as a student in the anatomy lab in the mid-60s was named "Linoleum." He explained that she had been given this name because she was an elderly black woman and it was his tablemates' speculation that she had earned her living in close proximity to other peoples' floors. This dynamic seems not to be one of humanization. Rather it seems to reflect the use of language and humor to whittle down the awesomeness and make the entire prolonged occasion more pleasant.

Student: "He's so fat it served him right he died."
Instructor: "We all do sometime."

This comment was made exuberantly by a male student on the second day of dissection. It was clearly intended to be humorous, but the garb of humor did not entirely cover the hostility. The instructor replied soberly to check the student's ungenerous judgement. Perhaps present here as well is the attempt to connect the observed fat with the cadaver's current state of affairs: it is always reassuring in medical work to encounter a cause of death which does not pertain to one's own situation.

> One student walked from his lab room into the next carrying a large square of skin surrounding the anus, carefully dissected away from his cadaver. As he marched into the room he asked loudly, "Does anyone want to see my asshole?"

Humor such as this is sensitive and uncomfortable to behold. Outside the moment of the joke we sit uncomfortably with such humor, and perhaps for this reason it goes largely unacknowledged. In fact, the examples cited here exemplify a great deal of laboratory humor that appears suddenly, inspires rapid laughter, and disappears.

It is in the nature of this sort of humor that tension is reduced specifically by minimizing or trivializing the experience at hand. Names given to cadavers suggest a class of people who die more frequently than the students' family or friends. "Gertrudes" or "Elmers" can easily be imagined as coming from a different world, ignorant and inept in matters of living, and perhaps poor as well. That their incompetence or poverty may have hastened their death is a comforting idea; it permits the antithesis of *identification* with them.

Even if one were to hold the content of lab humor insignificant, one would still be left to account for its sheer density per unit time. It was common during the three-hour lab session to hear bursts of laughter from adjacent tables within seconds of one another, or even simultaneously. Rapid bursts of laughter created a general sense of levity, and this in turn spawned further joking. The adaptive "antidepressant" function of the humor is greatly enhanced by its pace and density: laughter keeps things light. On many afternoons the din and hilarity inside could be heard as one approached the heavy black door from the outdoor stairs. It sounded like nothing so much as a lively party.

Student Dreams

The observations I have presented so far deal with public behavior. They are intriguing in their own right, but in order to understand them fully they must be seen in conjunction with students' private responses during the same period of time. To see if the idea of an unseen, internal student response makes sense, dream material gathered from the students of one class during the first month of anatomy will now be considered. Ten typical dreams will be presented here, accompanied by the dates they occurred.

October 2: "My mother was dead but she was still walking around. I was crying because she was dead. She kept saying that she didn't know what she was going to do now." The night the student had this dream he remembered opening his set of bones and recalling the line from Hamlet, "Alas, Poor Yorick!"

October 6: There was a killer in town and my life was endangered. A long and involved plot permeated by the theme of revenge. Thought of anatomy lab immediately upon awakening and felt that the dream was definitely instigated by the first day in the lab.

October 9: I was in a hospital for some reason when the Supreme Court made a decision which made me a criminal. Pursued ceaselessly for the entire length of this long dream, but in the end the Court reversed its decision and set me free. [In the midst of this long chase, the student's only refuge was offered by the kindly dean for student affairs.]

October 9: I took possession of a hand gun, and was accosted by a powerful crazed man. I imagined that he was attacking me so I shot him and killed him. Later in the dream I killed a frail white-haired man coming towards me with an outstretched palm. He had scared me. At the close of the dream another medical student persuaded me to give up the gun and turn myself over to the police.

October 8th: An escape artist was performing underwater with dangerous serpents. In the final trick the serpents would not let go and strangled me.

October 15: My parents told me that my grandmother had died several days before.

Students often commented that the cadavers evoked parents or grandparents, and that the experience of lab was an unwelcome reminder that parents eventually die.

October 20: I was home watching my own body; it had no face, no skin. My father was operating on me. Later, he went out to work on the car.

October 22: A friend told me that her friend's father had died.

October 22: I was dying of liver cancer.

October 24: I sat down at a greasy spoon type diner and ordered a cadaver.

This dream was so disturbing to the dreamer that the account, written down in October, was handed in to the observer in December.

A major theme reflected in students' more vivid dreams was the violation of important taboos regarding the dead. Findings in this study that students' dreams partially reflect a concern with violating the integrity of the dead bodies match James Knight's[1] anecdotal accounts of student dreams from their anatomy lab days. One of Knight's students dreamt that he was passing a haunted house with a cemetery in the front yard. While walking by, "fully dressed ashen gray bodies lifted themselves from the grave plots and swooped down [upon him]." He beat them back and ran.

One student, previously cited, spoke of a waking awareness of the theme of the cadavers' revenge. A reserved young man who prided himself on his well-controlled emotions, he reported that he counted the numbers of medical students and cadavers when he was in the lab at night. Though embarrassed by this silly idea, he admitted that he did this in case there was some sort of "uprising."

The second major theme of the students' dreams involved an awareness of personal mortality or the mortality of family or close friends. Frequently a dream would combine a student's father or mother with the anatomy under study. While studying the heart, a student might dream about a mother's anginal chest pain, or about a father's coronary bypass operation. Many students dreamed of re-experiencing an old injury or sickness, of being told that they had some dread illness, or of the death of parents or grandparents.

The following more detailed dream account, accompanied by the student's own associations, illustrates how dreams may be constructed out of the anatomy lab experience assembled with past events of personal significance:

> Everyone was in lab with the assignment to "work on" their own body. Each student was both dissector and specimen. I was replacing two body parts, the quadriceps [thigh] muscle and the phrenic nerve [to the diaphragm]. I made a quadriceps muscle out of wood; then I replaced the phrenic nerve with dental floss. The dream ended frighteningly when Dr. B. [the student's favorite

instructor] told me it would never work and predicted a grave outcome.

When asked about the significance of that specific thigh muscle, the student recalled a serious football injury in high school caused by a collision with another player. He remembered too that he was studying woodworking during that same semester, so that both problem and solution were drawn from his senior year of high school. His associations to the phrenic nerve led to breathing, and from breathing to his father living on the East Coast. The student had just been informed that his father had been awakening at night short of breath.

The associative link to the frailties and vulnerabilities of both self and parents was common in both dreams and waking thoughts. Nor should this be especially surprising. The facts of death and aging can be made abstract, put out of sight, or translated into symbol, but typically we do not dwell upon them for long. For some students, the confrontation with the dead body in lab simply links up with what has previously been repressed or actively excluded from consciousness. Repressed anxiety does not usually penetrate waking awareness, but here the experiential stimulus is too evocative to support the adaptive status quo entirely. Equilibrium is undermined and bad memories or fearful anticipations come to the fore in dreams, as if hooked or dredged from the unconscious by the sights of dissection.

Acute Stress Reactions

During my first two years of observing in the lab and speaking to students about their dreams and private thoughts, I became aware of a group of ten students who had an especially strong response to their time in lab. These students came to me either to share their dream reports or because they were "having trouble." I was struck by the intensity of their difficulty and, later, impressed by the resemblance of these vignettes to other accounts of acute psychological trauma.

Student one reported the occurrence of uncontrolled visual images while performing routine daily activities. Normal patterns of eating and sleeping were interrupted, and she regularly had unusually disturbing dreams. She began to worry about her health, and the visual images became associated with those fears. She would see, involuntarily, the image of the inside of her heart replete with anatomic detail. This image would be followed by palpitations and the fear that her heart might stop beating. She became preoccupied with the fragility of the body. She tried to speak to her tablemates in lab but found them uninterested: "they seemed to act like I was crazy." In one of several disturbing dreams she was carrying a severed head up an embankment in a coffee can when a bloodied facial bone popped up from the can. In another dream she was standing in waist-high river water as several cadavers floated by.

The second student who reported symptoms of acute stress experienced marked anxiety, insomnia, and periods of depression during the first few weeks of anatomy, but was also most troubled by intrusive visual images which she could not stop. These unbidden images would bring to mind some aspect of the lab experience which she found distasteful or frightening: "I would be brushing my teeth and would see pieces of skin." During the acute phase of the response she had great difficulty memorizing course material and these disturbing experiences dominated her life outside the lab. Gradually, the intensity of these reactions abated and life returned towards normal, though in January her distress reappeared in milder form with the dissection of the head and neck.

During the first weekend of the course student three experienced a sudden depressed state, began crying a lot, felt hopeless, and began ruminating about the meaning of life and about his own eventual death. In one nightmare he looked on as pallbearers carried his coffin.

During the dissection of the head and neck another student dreamt that her own head had been dissected off by fellow students who could now see down her neck and inside her body. This dream was followed by insomnia, bouts of crying, and melancholy which lasted about two weeks. During this time she experienced intrusive visual images, was reluctant to come to lab, and was unable to learn course material with any effectiveness, owing largely to an inability to concentrate.

Others of the ten students comprising this larger group had similar experiences, but each was unique, and in some the predominant symptom was an altered mood, while in others the sleep or dream disturbances were predominant. One student, for example, did not complain of intrusive visual images, but instead

	Intrusive images	Nightmares	Depression/ anxiety	Sleep	Memory
1	+	+	+	+	+
2	+	+	+	+	+
3	+	+	+	+	
4		+	+	+	
5		+	+	+	+
6	+	+	+	+	+
7		+	+	+	+
8		+	+	+	
9		+	+	+	+
10		+	+	+	

FIGURE 1

reported an extreme degree of hypochondriasis centered around the fear of contracting malignant disease from his cadaver.

"Post Traumatic Stress Disorder (PTSD)," the modern designation for what used to be termed "Traumatic Neurosis," is defined in the following way:

> The essential feature is the development of characteristic symptoms following a psychologically traumatic event that is generally outside the range of usual human experience. The characteristic symptoms involve re-experiencing the traumatic event; numbing of responsiveness to, or reduced involvement with, the external world; and a variety of autonomic, dysphoric, or cognitive symptoms. (DSM III, 1980)

Figure 1 illustrates the occurrence of these experiences in the group of ten students.

These vignettes, and the accompanying figure, demonstrate the close qualitative similarity between the experiences of a small group of medical students and the more intense clinical syndrome of PTSD. Although intrusive visual images and memory loss were not present in all of the students, nightmares, sleep disturbance, and altered mood were invariably present.

Although these ten vignettes represent no more than 5% of the total number of students observed in the larger study, their very existence suggests that emotions aroused by this experience can be stronger, and can create more of an internal management problem for the individual, than is generally conceded. For all of these students, the extent of their distress was unknown to the teaching faculty when it was most intense. This was not because of the faculty's unwillingness to deal with such concerns, but was rather due to the students' perceptions that such responses were unacceptable in this social setting.

The psychodynamic situation observed within the acute stress reactions was similar to that noted in relation to dreams earlier. Specifically, the sights and experiences of lab stirred up old fears and sadnesses and brought them to the surface, even after many years had passed. One student was reminded of devastating sights of war in Southeast Asia, another of the death of a parent. At least two students were reminded of the violent deaths of siblings.

Other students, not among this original group of ten, had similar dreams:

> One young woman had lost a sister in an automobile accident several years earlier. In her nightmares she would search for a grave or coffin, in images borrowed from both real life and the lab experience. In one especially harrowing dream the search ended with her discovery that the cadaver was her sister.

It may be that the severity of students' responses depends largely upon the nature of personal hardships endured or forgotten, but without the powerful reminder offered up by the dissection, such memories would likely lie dormant.

CONCLUSION

The student's response to emotional challenge goes on concurrently in several dimensions, some public, some private. Humor and horseplay, both public, must be interpreted because they do not reveal their meanng straightforwardly. Of course, first-year medical students do not often faint, choke, or rush from the room. This is not sufficient proof of psychic uneventfulness. The emotional or mental event is simply taken out of public view; it is either rendered private or is woven into everyday life in camouflaged form. Such adaptive transformations combine with the norms of concealment, and, together, they help account for the absence of brash signs of strained adjustment, here in the anatomy lab, and perhaps in the medical work world altogether.

The setting exposes students to potent psychological stimuli: the forced violation of very serious taboos about the dead body, and the vivid visual reminder of aging and the end of life. Students' explicit requirement is to learn the facts of anatomy. The faculty expends considerable effort at this responsibility. Students' emotional responses are assumed to be negligible. At the same time, certain traditions of conduct obtain in the lab proper, and these include the possibility of much talk and a great deal of laughter.

If we look closely at the laughter we can see that a major portion of it depends upon reducing the status of the cadaver to one that is less human, or at times even UNhuman. Dehumanization is a useful response. It lessens the impact of the experience. The meaning of the act, the experience, is changed when the cadaver is reassigned to the less-than-human.

In addition to normal everyday speech among classmates, the talk of lab contains the formal talk of anatomy texts and manuals, and the informal talk of med student bravado. In either case, tender or anxious feelings have no outlet. Concerns about death, about aging, about pain, have no place in this discourse.

The behavior of students in the lab reveals an inclination toward treating the body as material. It is the behavioral analogue to the rough language of "hacking and whacking." At odd moments the ironic awareness of how strange the situation is may be detected in humor or act, but for the most part the strangeness of the activity is never directly mentioned.

Such a view demands that evidence be brought forward to attest to the real difficulty inherent in this task: is there any indication of what lies deep to the everyday behavior of students? Is it truly something "hard to handle" or have we misread these observations of activity and humor?

In every major psychological system, there is agreement that dreams reflect shunted-aside or excluded mental contents. Both Jungians and Freudians agree that information and emotion embedded in the dream is often that which has been excluded from waking consciousness. Students in this study reported intense and unpleasant dreams that were unusual for them. The dreams frequently had as their focus the illness or death of student or loved one. Students who joked by day often had bad dreams or even nightmares at night. In talking about their dreams they would often talk about other concerns. In large numbers they admitted being bothered by the laboratory, or having their thoughts turn to illness and death more often than was comfortable.

Beyond the dreams and subjective accounts of students, we have evidence here that a small group of students has a profound psychological response that is well beyond what they have anticipated, and well beyond what has been anticipated for them by the faculty. This response attests to the intensity of the laboratory experience.

In order to begin a rational approach to medical training, educators will need to enlarge their understandings of what happens to students in the lab. Information about the real psychological experiences of student-physicians needs to become part of how we conceptualize both the anatomy lab and other experiences in medical training where powerful stimuli are paired with norms of silence.

REFERENCE

1. James A. Knight, *Medical Student: Doctor in the Making,* New York: Appleton-Century-Crofts, 1973.

Sorcerer's Apprentice:
Memoirs of a Medical Student

John A. McKinnon

I

The first-year medical student is a self-conscious, unprepossessing creature: more man-on-the-street than physician, more ignorant and unable than he ever will be again, he is an eager, nervous neophyte, an incompetent in a white coat. And this white coat is his paradox and riddle, expressing a wish and a promise but not yet the reality of "physician."

It is conventional wisdom that a physician is a person in a long white robe who heals the sick, walks on water, and makes enough bread to feed a multitude. In contradistinction, civilians, i.e., patients, are ignorant and precariously mortal creatures who don't. There remains, between these clear extremes, confusion. For, neither fish nor fowl, traditionally poor as a churchmouse and yet privileged in some ways like a physician, what is a medical student? There was no clear answer for me this year, and so the year's toil in the classroom and even its moments of conceptual clarity occurred in a sunlit foreground. In the background shadows slouched this unsettling ambiguity.

This chapter began as four memoirs written at the end of each of the author's years in medical school (1972–75) and published in the Case Western Reserve University *Medical Alumni Bulletin*. More than a decade later the author has cut length and clarified sense, but has tried to restrain the natural impulse of age to revise the past.

The first-year's memoir, "A Neophyte's Notes on the Rites of Initiation" was republished in *WHO Dialogue OMS*, Magazine of the Geneva Staff, World Health Organization, April 1973. Excerpts from all four were published as the cover story in *The New Physician*, November 1977.

Surely this role ambiguity is not solely to do with medical incipience. Men and women entering other professions endure a transitional period during which they gradually come to identify themselves with the role. And the rites of medical initiation seem to work; we began to think of ourselves as physicians and stopped gaping when someone called us "doctor." But I doubt the novices in any other profession, morticians and strippers being exceptions, endure so shifting a conception and so extreme an awareness of their own bodies or so radical a revision of taboos. Here we learn to speak in a new jargon about four-letter events, now without giggles.

The process of making the external image of physician an integral part of our conceptions of ourselves seemed to begin with the short white clinic coat. Around these coats surfaced an agitated, tedious, but otherwise likeable worry over fraudulence and also both defiance and compromise attempts at integrity, all of which reflected the gap we sensed between what we knew we were and what the white coat signified to us: the physician's role. No doubt first-year students every year again feel the same concern that patients will be "fooled" by the white coat, that they may unwittingly allow the impostor to do or to hear what he would not otherwise be permitted, and that we were invading a privacy without hope of contributing to the patient's care. These concerns were the more troubling when the patients "fooled" are black and poor, and when we suspect this segment of the population bears a responsibility for educating physicians that will not be fully reciprocated.

But be that as it may, I did not share the enthusiasm of some of my classmates for shedding the coat altogether, nor for rushing to inform patients of my irrelevance to their care, nor for establishing friendships instead of professional relations. For it seemed to me that while such "integrity" served well the conscience of the student, it failed to make the patient more secure. We have to see medicine practiced if we are to become competent, ourselves, and I cannot imagine a patient wanting a man-off-the-street, much less a "friend," to witness his proctoscopic exam, or hear his history. The medium (the white coat) must convey the message of a purely professional interest. And so I thought I had to learn to wear it.

And in time, the fraud began to seem less blatant. It was in part a function of knowing something, although many times sick patients looked up at me with a hushed respect and willingness to confess all that otherwise they reserved for their Makers and confided in graphic detail just how their bowels were or were not working, and for all the instrumental good I could do them they might as well have confided in the janitor. But the masquerade taught me what the receiving end of That Look feels like and, after a time, how to shape my bearing so as to reassure, to comport myself in such a way, with an understanding smile and knowing nod, that the patient knows his constipation is part of a benign process of fate whose outcome I have been given to know in advance. Thus, inasmuch as this idealization of the doctor always involves distortion of the truth, there is an element of "fraud" anytime a physician permits it. And so the "masquerade" turns out not to be just a matter of pretending to be a doctor, but part of becoming one, of feeling like one, of enduring the transference.

But patients don't just idealize physicians. Some of the most ghoulish, nightmarish creatures of the popular and literary mind are doctors: Faustus, Jekyll, Caligari, Mengele. One source of this fascination, I think, is the transgression of our culture's central and strict taboos regarding death and the human body. Frankenstein's monster is an animated hodgepodge of body parts filched from the dissecting room, and reassembled in an epic organ transplantation. I need not belabor the point. No doubt the depth of feeling which corpses, disease, dismemberment, surgery, and the rest of it evoke is the counterpart of the conscious adulation and awe physicians enjoy. The doctor is both loved and hated, needed and dreaded. These possibilities need to be remembered when reflecting upon medical education, for the ordeal of initiation in medical school involves the violation of taboos, and the students who come to medicine are as influenced as anyone else by tales of sacred miracle cures, and of Jekyll and Hyde, and Frankenstein.

Naturally we anticipated facing down a corpse, for this is traditional. But I was startled, anyway. I remember the day a student opened one of the unobtrusive metal refrigerators that line the back of the lab in which for two months we had been working, unaware we were not alone. Inside lay a shrouded supine figure, a pale leg protruding from under the damp white sheets. It was a moment whose excitement we did our best to hide from one another. A month later we began our ritual dissection, without the grotesque horsing around with the cadavers I had dreaded, but nonetheless had expected. We were to all appearances just intellectually interested in where the kidneys lie and what the aorta connects to. But we were confronting our human frailty, too, or at least strong evidence of it. At night I dreamed of pallid cotylidons sprouting from the earth.

And if the dissections were assaults on a social ban, there were other experiences with living subjects which introduced us to the violent, invasive aspects of medicine. I suppose the Family Clinic obstetric experience was the most evocative, in part because it occurred early in the year and also because it was so powerfully sexual. The focus of unrest and concern was the pelvic exam, and I lost track of the number of lunchtime discussions which responded to the question: "Would you want medical students doing pelvic examinations on you (your girlfriend, your wife, your mother, your grandmother, etc)?" This particular examination is, of course, a particularly powerful symbol, but only one extreme in a spectrum of more or less assaultive, humiliating, intrusive examinations and procedures. This was the lesson: it's *all* an assault on taboos, *all* intrusive. Done with the patient's consent and with his express wish, medical and surgical and psychiatric examinations are never permitted without ambivalence or done without feeling. Even excitement.

And given this, I saw that most of us came to clinical medicine in part because we were fascinated to penetrate, to intrude behind the bounds of privacy, because we are fascinated by death, pain, blood, the whole drama. These are not the incidentals to medicine, but rather the fundamental spectacle. At the very least they are the conditions under which we have chosen to view our fellow man for most of the waking hours of the rest of our lives. It will be under these stresses that we will be witness to the dignity, courage, kindness, or lack of these qualitites, in our patients. I might have missed this about myself and about my classmates, if I had not noticed how assiduously we sought these spectacles in a year of training not particularly concerned with clinical medicine. I myself attended post-mortems, spent evenings on the preemie service at Babies and Childrens, watched surgery, attended elctro-convulsive therapy sessions at Hanna Pavillion, and I still rise at 5:45 to draw blood on the wards. And when I go there, I find my classmates.

This should be no surprise. For they and I are caught up in the same curiousity about how the body works, the same fascination with how the person reacts when the body does not work, which has always brought students to medicine. The man or woman, their diseases, surgery, pain, fear, feces, urine and blood, and, in the end, their deaths, are magnets to a Faustian curiousity we share. Its ultimate object is ourselves.

II

For me the second year was a dry time in a dry lab. After the novelties of the first year—anatomy lessons, Family Clinic patient, white coat, morning blood to draw—the second year was anticlimax: frequent examinations, but much the same. My Family Clinic patient, now familiar, remained, and I saw her in my short white coat, now frayed from washing. In the dawn the sleepy patients no longer called me "you damned fool," for in the narrow defile of the antecubital fossa, I knew where I was. And if that weren't all, my cadaver grew mold over the summer; its parched tissues disgusted me. In short, I greeted them all that second September with a dried-up enthusiasm. I was impatient to get to the wards.

Fortunately I had an old friend, two years ahead of me, to assure me that I would often feel bored, and that this *ennui* itself would become familiar. He warned me there would be days when kidney physiology would seem prosaic, when good intentions would not prevent clinical sleep at the very mention of Group A streptococci. "Just relax," he said. "Watch a John Wayne movie on the tube, or read *Light in August*, or take your wife to the museum or to bed (where she's been going alone these many months)." He called this kind of hiatus "Waiting for Rain," and he told me that soon, and sooner if I followed his prescription, I would begin to feel restless to get back to the books. The dry weather would pass.

During this year such moments of boredom came and went. It seemed a year of "waiting for rain," and I was grateful for the advice, which I took.

* * *

Family Clinic had introduced me to Ms. B, who was 22 and pregnant, in my first year. From the first months of our mutual need she treated me with a formality which, although it came to be cordial, never significantly changed over the two years. In that period of changing physicians, obstetricians, and social workers, my face remained the constant ornament, such as it was, in her experience with University Hospitals. I did that much for her. During those interminable hours of her lonely induced labor at MacDonald House she realized I was stubborn, determined to stick it, and over the next year she acknowledged this fact of life by an increased respect and trust.

Since I was privy to her situation at home, did her physical exams with my preceptor and attended her baby's every rash, she saw no reason to pretend with me. Nonetheless, she didn't know quite what to call me. She couldn't pretend she believed me a physician, so she didn't call me "doctor," but on the other hand, I wasn't "mister," either. Consequently, for about a year she avoided calling me anything at all. I came to be amused by her dilemma, since it was essentially my own, and I waited for the situation to corner her. Finally she had to call me at home, and she spoke first with my wife, asking for "John." Since we were cordial by this time, I thought the matter settled. But to my face she still avoided my name, and then, somewhere in our second year together, she taught me the subtlety of the situation when, in the waiting room, she introduced me to a friend as "Dr. McKinnon." She had no need with my wife, or with me, to protect my dignity or her own, but before an "outsider," she dignified our situation.

Clinic visits involved the well-being of L, the new arrival, whose first year and a half caused me less anxiety than the prenatal period had. L developed a healthy hatred for me, for my white coat and prying fingers and cold steel, and her early development explicated the text. From her I inferred the pediatric corollary to Newton's Law, which is: "Well babies tend to stay well." I had so little of interest to report to my preceptor group in L's first year of life that I was driven, just to keep from boring them, to teasing about her faulty, but promising, blank verse. In this there was an oddly paternal pride. In any case, I got no rise from the other students, whose patients had problems so monumental by comparison.

In the happy course of things, L's clinic visits became fewer, further between, and Ms. B and I saw one another infrequently. In the Spring, in anticipation of the end that comes to all things, she produced a camera and snapped her squirming daughter perched on her student-doctor's lap. At our final visit she presented me a copy of that photograph of my first pediatric patient, and then she took her daughter's hand, shook mine, and the two of them walked out of my life without any of us letting go that formality we had sustained against all indignity. But not without feeling.

* * *

The arrival of the new first-year students produced instant seniority of a paltry kind, reminding me that I had learned something the prior year. Their polite inquiries as to where the men's and lady's rooms were permitted us all to relish the fact we knew more than *someone*, and all too ephemerally they sat at our feet, avid gratifying consumers of our Mayfly wisdom. In these months I heard (and delivered) countless lectures on housing, on Family Clinic and preferred textbooks, on bad faculty lecturers and the other cadavers, and for a time we were happy experts. Briefly we dictated the commercial habits and first frame of mind of the class of '76. But it didn't last. The new students learned all too soon that seniority does not guarantee good judgment, only advanced age. Shortly we were left alone again to endure the tedium of the now entirely predictable class routine.

And in this year the curriculum does become predictable. This was, in a way, its relief and its point: to teach that the ways the body becomes sick are not infinite! The process is like bird-watching. First I was like a man who knows nothing about birds and keeps saying, "Look, there's one with a yellow tail and a beak like a tweezers!" In the face of this ignorance, which is not unlike Adam's, the possibilities seem endless, without name or rhyme or reason. But the experienced bird-watcher is less intimidated, and so is the second-year medical student. I began to see there are only a finite number of ways the body or its organs become sick. I learned this by tedious repetition, but in the end I saw what all physicians come to think of as a firm grasp of the obvious: that while the basic knowledge required is enormous, it is not infinite! Like Adam, I began to spot again some of the ones I'd already given a name to: familiar facts, analogous patterns, yet another use for a familiar drug.

This dawning first grasp of the broad field was meant to come together in time for Part I of the National Board Examinations in Medicine. Naturally there was anxiety among us, despite faculty who belittled its importance. We knew it wasn't important so long as we didn't fail it! And so toward the end of the year some students who'd slept through lectures with astonishing regularity began to skip class and to read books. And early apostates, who'd not been seen for months at the daily sermons, began to show up with the zeal of converts, afraid to miss the good word.

And then the exams—or more accurately the beer and pretzel party which followed—brought the class together for the last time until graduation. There was much loud laughter, noisy talk about how stupid the exam had been, and, as I remember, an early and acute shortage of beer. Then came diaspora, the clinical assignments around the city which would force us to study different problems and to learn different clinical languages in different places. In one of those chance encounters which became for me the paradigmatic meeting for members of the third- and fourth-year classes, I asked an acquaintance what he had to say about the second year. We were picking up white trousers for clerkships at Metropolitan General Hospital, meeting in the sub-basement. He turned to go back up to Medicine as I set off for Obstetrics, and, hoisting his laundry onto his shoulder, he said: "Let's get ON with it! I'm glad as hell it's over!" I was, too.

III

The dense mass of the third-year clerkships resists brief description. The time consumed would require two years in any ordinary job, and the diversity of Medicine, Psychiatry, OB-GYN, Surgery, and

Peds makes any generalization crude. Therefore, hoping to make these elliptical notes stand for the whole, I shall concentrate upon my first experience of Medicine, and a few of the events that changed me for good and for the better.

Even leaving aside my global initial incompetence at the simplest practical medical tasks—naso-gastric tubes and Foleys, lumbar punctures, blood gases, blood smears and stains, urine dip-sticks and microscopic—there was a more fundamental trans-formation of abstract knowledge into tangible experience and personal memory. I knew a lot of anatomy and physiology and pathology, even at the start of the year, but yet I said over and over again, as the months went by: "So *that's* what it looks like!"

Having written that sentence, I immediately think of my first death. Before I started on 45 North, a woman's ward attached to the GI intensive care unit at University Hospitals, I knew alive persons, and I knew a few dead ones (cadavers), but I had never witnessed the transformation of the one into the other, this (like childbirth and parental sex) one of the ultimate taboo experiences, an event that happened behind closed doors, well beyond a line I certainly had never crossed.

Mrs. G was a handsome young woman a few years older than I, the mother of four children. She came late at night, admitted with a gastrointestinal hemorrhage, the patient of a prominent cardiac surgeon who aroused my envy and wounded my dignity when he asked me to move away while he talked in a low voice, intimately, with her. I could hear the "click-click" of her valve. She was endoscoped at about 1 a.m. Bright red blood painted the lavage tube, as her blood poured out into a pan. Good for nothing else, I cradled her head while the GI professor, immaculate in a white coat that remained forever without stain, sought her bleed's source with his black snake stuck down her throat, gagging her, its end twisting down inside her, lighting up her dark viscera (when I got a look) like downtown. Soon the sheets, the floor, and the resident's scrub shirt were spattered with blood, and the air stank.

Finally her bleeding stopped, and the GI staff went home, the nurses and the sheets changed, and the floor got mopped. In the quiet that settled over 45 North I returned to finish my work-up, feeling foolish and (rightly) that I was bothering her. She wanted to talk, however, and she wanted to hold my hand. Hers was clammy cold. There was a tube in her nose, a tube in her rectum, and both drained a slow stream of red. IVs punctured both arms, fresh blood in one, a yellow fluid in the other. Her chest was wired to the monitor, which bleated with every systole.

She was "sorry": sorry in a polite and unimportant way for my having to bother about her and because I was away from my wife; and profoundly sorry about "Hank and the children." But she was so wan and wasted and weary she seemed reconciled, except for the regret and the fear that kept her holding tightly onto my hand when she said "it's going to be tonight." I tried to sound confident, relaxed, sure of a benign outcome, and this wasn't so difficult, because I had never seen any other kind. But she only smiled a sad smile. She'd been in Intensive Care before, but this time was "different." She "wouldn't mind, but for Hank and my boys and my baby girl," who had "had to bear so much." Half naked, her skinny haunch exposed, too tired and inured to care, she looked slight and perhaps for that reason very young, suddenly: a scrawny grieving girl. She said then that she liked me, that my wife was lucky, and then she dozed. Alone in the residents' office, I fell asleep over my write-up.

I was wakened by a nurse speaking loudly near my ear and waving a monitor strip. I ran for the intern, who was in the shower. "Get 200 mg of Pronestyl ready," he said, and I ran out, feeling sort of important, but also ridiculous, since I wouldn't have recognized 200 mg of Pronestyl if it had materialized in my hand, and I surely didn't know how to tell if it was "ready." But the nurse did, and I was left to fidget at the bedside, self-conscious about not having anything to do, since the nurses bustled about the room, intent, sure of their role in the catastrophe they sensed coming, and ignoring me, or politely pretending not to notice my uselessness, the way one looks away from an embarrassing disability. I took Mrs. G's pulse, since that was one of the things I knew how to do, concentrating over that cold boney wrist until it dawned on me I could hear her heartbeat from across the room, her valve now going "clickety-clack-clack" in a new way. Then the alarm on the monitor went off, and the intern burst through the door. I was probably gaping at the monitor screen, which looked like a bleak horizon at sea.

"She's flat-line!" he said. "Hit her, you big clown!" I smashed her boney chest with my fist and leaned over her sternum, pumping as I'd been shown, while the intern attended to her airway and, outside in the empty, pre-dawn corridor, that nasal disembodied voice intoned: "The Anesthetist, The Anesthetist, The Anesthetist, 45 North." The Chief Resident came in to preside at the EKG, and the room began to fill with white coats. Men and women who knew what they were doing shouldered me aside, attending to gases, injecting drugs into her IV, and shocking her. Mrs. G's neck was craned backwards, her eyes wide open in an unblinking stare, and with every pumping thrust her frail body jerked. The surgeon came in, looked at the EKG, and making the melodramatic gesture her extremity invited and excused, he climbed onto the bed and, bending over her, shoved a six-inch needle into her chest, injecting epinephrine directly into the right ventricle.

It had been half an hour. No spontaneous heartbeat. Her pupils were fixed, dilated. The surgeon exchanged a glance with the Chief Resident and subtly nodded. "OK people," the Chief Resident said. And everyone stood away. The scrawny woman lay still, and I stared at her while the others filed out, shrugging their shoulders and returning to interrupted conversations. Finally I went out. In the corridor the intern caught up with me and proposed, brightly, that I grab a laryngoscope and practice putting down an endotracheal tube, using her body. "Best way to learn," he said, shrugging when I looked away. In the cafeteria I smiled and waved to acquaintances. I found my wife and put my back to the room and unexpectedly, just as I began importantly to tell her about my exciting night, I started to cry.

* * *

I took the nine assembled relatives of a comatose Mrs. W into a conference room and explained her profound congestive failure to them. After that, I was "the doctor," and no explanation about my low status and clinical unimportance in her care made any impression. When I left for the day, her brothers, standing sentry duty in the hall outside the ICU, shook my hand and asked if I'd given the intern "[my] orders?" In the morning when I returned, family replacements now on duty expressed satisfaction I was "back on the job."

Mrs. W, herself, was a cardiac mess. She'd been shocked some eighty times, and her myopathy, having thinned the walls of her heart, blowing it up like a balloon, kept trying to kill her. And so she was on a respirator, had a Foley up into her bladder, and IV's in both arms. I fussed over her eletrolytes and gasses, helping the resident in what looked like an elaborate metabolic experiment.

But while the resident stayed calm, interested only in her kidneys and in teasing me about "my" patient, I fell for this comatose, supine woman whose chest we'd burned with our shock paddles. I talked about her constantly, badgering the intern about her electrolytes, reporting her progress to my wife, and keeping her family informed and encouraged. I talked to her as I worked around her bed, thinking she might be able to hear, and implicitly I gave her a pleasing personality. Moreover, without fully knowing I was doing so, I imagined her smiling, tearfully profuse thanks when, recovered, this saintly wife and sister left me in a haze of gratitude and good feeling to go back to her doting family.

But all good things must end, and one day she stirred and woke up. By the end of a week, even before she'd been extubated, I could no longer hide from myself my intense dislike of her. In brief, she was demanding, spoiled, complaining, selfish, and lacking in courage. She resisted every procedure, cussed her nurse and doctor and medical student, and she had a very dirty mouth. The intern said she was "too mean to die." Naturally I was teased. And so I was relieved when my rotation soon ended, that I might slink away.

* * *

A delightful 80-year-old black woman from Mississippi, Mrs. M, whose accent and insistence upon calling me "sir" reminded me of her origins every time she spoke to me, was admitted with "black stools," and I, puffed up with the confidence one only feels after doing something four times without serious mishap, helped a second-year student, a friend visiting me on the ward, to put the needed nasogastric tube down. He did it pretty well, all things considering, especially given that Mrs. M prayed noisily all the while that Sweet Jesus might vouchsafe an explanation for this apparently gratuitous torment of a true-believer and, while He was at it, that He might forgive us in His mercy, for clearly we knew not what we were doing. When we had finished, she thanked us sincerely and very kindly for our trouble and apologized for making such a racket. This was my violent introduction to her, but we had other less complicated talks over the next days as I helped work her up for what seemed likely (given the X-rays) to be cancer of the stomach.

Three days after admission I was called abruptly from rounds to see her, just back from the X-rays I had written orders for. "Please hurry!" the nurse said. I found her unresponsive on the gurney, both pupils dilated, and as I examined her, she wasn't breathing and her pulse stopped. There was a "code," and we all did our best, but much of the paltry scene I described above repeated itself, including its ending. She was pronounced dead within the hour.

I mention this death not simply out of sentimentality, but because the autopsy that I persuaded her assembled Cleveland children and grandchildren to permit revealed she had died of "spinach wedged firmly in both mainstem bronchi." I don't know how that spinach got there, although I suppose the possibilities are obvious enough. In any case, she did not die from the benign stomach polyps which caused her "black stools." She died of "morbidity and mortality" associated with hospitalization and tests, and I am now unable to order a "routine" upper G̅I̅ series without remembering Mrs. M, who prayed for us, and how she died of institutional spinach.

IV

Most sane medical students did not spend time their final year as acting interns. Their actual internships would soon enough suffice for them. Instead they spent their fourth years on specialty services, without night call, seeing consults and reading, sharpening their technical knowledge free from the daily responsibility of direct care.

The acting intern, by contrast, is a senior student who rashly volunteers for night call every third day and the grinding, sleepless routine of the intern. He reports more or less directly to the resident, carries the intern's load of admissions and inpatients, dictates the same charts, fills out the same lab slips, and leaves unread the same books and journals. The differences include: no salary (and instead the university bill for tuition); less experience and a less official status and therefore greater anxiety; and both the excitement of a child stepping into a grown-up's shoes and the necessary indignity of having to have even the simplest order counter-signed before a nurse could accept it.

It's a little hard to acknowledge the excitement and fright of those first nights of responsibility. Most experienced physicians, even residents, carry this burden with such grace that the observer is not even aware of it, nor are physicians themselves. They rapidly forget the weight of that monkey, and perhaps it is only during those first weeks while that monkey climbs up and settles its haunches, hunkering down for a lifetime, that its mass and heft are fully felt. Certainly now my responsibilities are far greater, but I no longer feel them the way I did during my acting internship.

I began in January, 1974, on a general medical ward of 42 patients, whose front-line care would normally be divided among three interns, supported and supervised by a resident, who answered in turn to a Chief Resident and to a staff Visitant, who would finally answer to the courts and presumably to his Maker. On this ward, however, there were two interns, because the hired third one had arrived, had taken one look, climbed back onto the Rapid, and rushed to the airport to fly away. The two remaining interns were more than glad to share their outsized burden with me, and by the end of the first week I was taking night call alone on the ward every third night, the resident "float" covering four such units available to sign my orders and to help in a crisis.

But otherwise that sleeping ward was my problem, and that first night the monkey arrived and settled in for the duration. It was an uneventful night, I think. We held sign-out rounds, and the other interns and the resident posted me on problems I might expect, and then they left, calling the intern's farewell: "Hope you get some sleep!" I checked the beeper, and waited. I think I had an admission. One patient couldn't sleep, another had pain, and one nice lady was worried in the middle of the night about her immobile bowels. These were the only ripples that disturbed my pond.

But I was so excited I found even these small problems exhilarating to solve, and the fact I knew how to solve them, all by myself, was an enormous relief. I sat alone in the cramped, windowless ward office reading through charts, waiting for some catastrophe to test my mettle, rehearsing the moves I would make when "IT" happened, and I never got my clothes off, never slept. I went to the on-call room, a dismal four walls and bed with no window but with a lightswitch, a toilet, a sink and shower and, connecting me to the ward just down the hall, a telephone whose ominous presence made it feel like trying to sleep beside a ticking package. I stared at the dark ceiling for hours, my eyes snapped wide open, demonstrating the impossibility of sleeping when you're holding your breath and starting at every noise.

But it turns out also to be impossible to stay awake during the day if your aren't sleeping at night! This statement may sound extreme to anyone who's not been awake for most of two or three days (and this experience is not common outside of medicine), but every intern knows it's true: that when you're *that* tired sleep becomes involuntary, a narcoleptic event, almost a seizure of dozing off, a sleep that happens to you rather than something you do. For example, sitting in the front row, literally toe-to-toe with the Chief of Medicine, I asked a question during rounds and fell asleep during the answer. I woke up in an empty classroom, trying to remember what happened. The Chief's only complaint later was about my snoring.

In the hospital I awoke and had the phone to my ear on the first ring, but on occasion at home I became psychotic when my wife tried to wake me up. With my eyes wide open, I would slam things around and shout, "No more! I'm too tired." After three cups of coffee and on the way down the hill in the car, I would cool off from my rage and apologize to my patient wife, but to my chagrin, it happened more than once. In fact, friends from another town once called when my wife was out for the evening, and I had fallen asleep on the living room floor. I gather I talked with them for some 15 minutes, but hadn't made any sense—I'd gone on and on about "gomers" (a contemptuous term I never use when awake), nurses, urine samples, NG tubes, and people they had never heard of. Despite their shouting over the line, I never did come awake, and their sad conclusion was that my wife had divorced me and I'd had a "nervous breakdown." This was off the mark, but not far enough to suit me.

For an intern's life strains a marriage to the snapping point at times. Wives or husbands of interns—whose conjugal relations are reduced to watching a spouse sleep or to talking on the phone at midnight; to enduring a partner's exhausted apathy or irritability; to listening with the wanted smile of interest plastered on and summoning the wanted admiration for an obsessive preoccupation that does not include them; to taking abuse displaced from where it rightly belongs (hospital, patients, demands); to a truncated social life and an empty bed (or good as) most nights for months on end—may be forgiven for thinking the medical stick short and their end dirty. Because it often is.

At my end, the stick got slippery, but holding onto it made much the same sense that swallowing goldfish or marching around Georgia at 2 a.m. have always made: those who endure pass the initiation trial and will earn membership in the fraternity, whether it's medicine or the 82nd Airborne. And enduring is more than getting let in on the secret handshake, more than learning to do a Gram stain or to field strip a weapon. The intern's trial seems necessary to a medical *esprit de corps*, an identification with the values of the medical fraternity. The resulting pride, the strong sense of physicianly integrity, and an exultant feeling of alienation from the rest of humanity, mark its efficacy. Given the privileges, rightly called, that go with the license to practice, this barrier, this trial, this primitive, emotion-laden inculcation of values probably makes a kind of social sense, albeit not an entirely logical kind of sense. I hated the fatigue and the strain of these months, but once I had endured it, I felt proud. I also feel a little silly for this pride, but I feel it, nonetheless.

The sense of triumph and privilege which ultimately sustains such otherwise irrational trials as an internship has something to do with "having *been* there" with a patient, with seeing the sights and hearing the sounds and smelling the odors and touching those otherwise private, taboo sights, sounds, smells, and bodily places to do with his suffering, his sexuality, his survivals, and his deaths. I sometimes asked myself as I walked away from the hospital on a sunny day and saw The Others getting on the bus, shopping, eating, or otherwise turning to their mundane tasks: "How many men have seen what I have seen, or heard or smelled what I have heard and smelled today?" And I remembered why I'm doing this, why I put up with it all, and why, in short, I'm gladly joining *this* fraternity.

It is easy in an almost immediately-writ-down memoir to dwell entirely on the traumatic failures and catastrophes, and I am going to record one more, but before doing so, it would be remiss not to mention the occasional triumph which lit up my personal sky. I think, for example, of Mr. L, who twice came to the acute care unit during my tenure there, each time with pulmonary edema and swollen in the extremitites with peripheral edema, his heart in failure and having stopped breathing in the ambulance. This Lazarus twice responded to my care and lived to slap my back and call me "Doc." He was not the only one. There were moments of feeling potent, however junior I was, feeling exhilerated to be alive and to be doing *this*!

And before going on to my final sad story, I should say that one of the gratifying lessons of the year was: "Patients *tend* to survive the inevitable mistakes." It's not that you *can't* kill them with an error, but rather that most of the errors personal ignorance, lack of sleep, over-work and lapses in judgment make inevitable the patient will do his or her best to survive. Only the negligence lawyer summing up his argument will insist that medicine must and even can be practiced without mistakes. As a more senior friend has told me: "Increasing competence does not imply a more arcane mistake, but rather making the simple mistakes less often." And so there *will* be doseage errors, times when the diagnosis which seems obvious in retrospect fails to get made in time, and when the failure to order the critical test or to call for help soon enough costs someone dearly. There *will*. But also, many times, the patient will survive the imperfect practice. For a beginning physician, who had worried, of course not without implicit hubris, that any imperfection in his thought and reflex would bring disaster, this lesson was, in part, welcome. Its corollary, a very old lesson in medicine, was not. It is: that no matter how smart you are, there are times when there is little to do except endure disaster.

A 23-year old wife and mother was transferred to the ICU in which I worked. Married only 15 months, she had a four-month-old daughter. Two days before she had arrived at another hospital's emergency room with complaints of urinary retention, but by the time she came to us she was becoming paralyzed from the neck down, and it was our business to get her on a respirator. Her paralysis had, on close questioning, probably proceeded from her fingers and toes toward her trunk, and we fixed upon the diagnosis of Guillain-Barre's radiculopathy. There was a lot of senior advice, and we settled her down (under my immediate, front-line care) to weather the storm, to provide respiratory and other supportive, watchful care until she spontaneously recovered and could walk out of the hospital to her family.

I felt some confidence about my part in this prognosis. This was the end of my year, and I was good at kidney physiology and knew, basically, how to manage someone on a respirator. I took her history from her husband and confirmed it, getting her to nod her head, and then I told him what to expect: weeks of waiting, our care about infection and respiratory problems, but because he looked so scared, I think, I all but promised him she would come home to him and their little girl. Then I explained to her, slowly, what she could expect, and she nodded her head and tried to smile.

Then, in mid-evening, things stopped adding up tidily. Her WBC was too high (25,000), her temperature soaring (to 106), the pattern of her sensory-motor loss less typical, suggesting a transverse myelitis, rather than Guillain-Barre. The resident was on the phone with the attending, and we were starting cortisone IV when all hell broke loose. The nurse couldn't get a blood pressure or a pulse, the patient's pupils were a full centimeter across, and suddenly she had become unresponsive. No heart sounds, no pulse. We began emergency resuscitation, another student pounding on her chest, and now there was frank red blood draining from her endotracheal tube and red blood draining vaginally. The temperature went off the end of the thermometer, and an ice blanket was rushed in. Her EEG was an omelette. And I thought: Good God, we're going to lose this lady, and I don't even know what in hell is going on!"

And so we did. And I spent the next two weeks wondering what I hadn't known, what I'd neglected to do, that would have saved her. I felt vulnerable, sick that the autopsy I'd talked her stricken husband into permitting would reveal my negligence, would demonstrate a curable problem I hadn't thought of. Late at night and intrusively during the day there seemed many candidates for this missed diagnosis.

But the last day of my acting internship I attended Mortality and Morbidity Rounds in which her case was discussed. The autopsy revealed, to my relief, a hemorrhagic necrosis of the entire neuroaxis white matter, brain and cord both, and emboli in both pulmonary arteries. In short, we hadn't, in our ignorance, missed something we could have cured. I stumbled into the Cleveland sunshine, queasy and uneasy still, the image of the death of this young mother and the look on the face of her husband that wretched morning vividly before me, and the memory of the promise I'd glibly offered him still raw.

I crossed to the medical school to attend a lecture for first-year students, because I was a preceptor in the clinical science program. When the lights went off for slides I immediately fell asleep, but I woke up while a few students were angrily accusing the staff physicians on a panel of "ripping off" patients in the clinic for their own selfish purposes, of racism and insensitivity, of cowardice, of exploiting the poor. And I suppose there may have been the same elements of truth there had been when I started medical school, but in four years something had changed. Watching these graying physicians, who were not debaters, trying to talk across that gulf of years and experience, struggling to explain themselves and what seemed to them their good intentions, I became very angry.

I had not slept, and I had this young dead woman on my mind, and it seemed to me then that some self-righteous nitwits who hadn't "been there" and with the luxury of a night's sleep were pointing the finger. And inasmuch as they pointed the finger of blame—entirely without irony—at imperfect practice, they were pointing that righteous, ignorant finger at me. I saw that a gulf of incomprehension had opened between us, probably late at night, when I was tired and trying to explain to a man why his wife wasn't going to come home to him. And looking around at these fresh, beginning students, I saw I was no longer one of them and couldn't be, ever again. I felt a little grieved, too, in the way that it's sad to discover you've grown up.

Notes from Overground:
Fourth Year at Harvard Medical School

Daniel J. Bressler

It is too late for first impressions and too early for memoirs, yet I want to try to leave some record of what I have learned in medical school. This is not an essay on electrolyte changes in chronic renal failure or the differential diagnosis of hemoptysis. Rather, it tells what one medical student gleaned incidentally, between the lines of the formal medical school instruction.

The last 3½ years have changed the way I think of myself. I have gone from considering myself a "layperson" to thinking of myself as a physician. Much of this transformation is related to the body of information I have been so busy accumulating—information that has allowed me to participate in decisions concerning the welfare and fate of my patients. But a large part of the change is due to my exposure to "medical" experiences rather than to the accumulation of bits of information. These experiences are not listed in the medical school syllabus.

Suddenly I have found myself privy to the underbelly and the hidden thoughts of humanity. A modest grandmother has shown me the skin lesion on her inner thigh. I have heard the secret fears of an old man that he would never tell his wife of 50 years. I have caught babes first squeezed out from their mothers' wombs and held them as they gasped their first breath. I have stayed up late reading Shakespeare with a man who had cancer and was trying his best to die cheerfully. I have stared into the blank face of a pretty teenaged girl who could not understand why she kept slitting her wrists and overdosing on barbiturates.

What is most remarkable about these tales of close encounters is how "unremarkable" they are. Every medical student has a handful of such images and meetings by the time of graduation. I lay out these memories not to claim some special experience for myself, but to point out the privileged eyes and ears we are given. Amidst the barrage of exams, evaluations, national boards, blood drawing, and emotional turmoil, it is easy to forget or grow numb to these privileged senses. But for few other people in society are the raw ingredients of life spread out so plainly in their beauty and ugliness. And on few others is the capacity to participate helpfully in another person's life bestowed so generously.

This is not meant as an *apologia* for the defects of the American system of medical education or the Harvard Medical School in particular. These institutions, rife with problems, are often impersonal and often operate under the burden of traditions that are no longer effective or meaningful. Harvard Medical School, in particular, is full of pretense and hierarchy. It is filled with ambition, a quality that often interferes with the softer attributes of kindness and compassion. Certainly, each of us could draw up our own bill of grievances. And yet, although new approaches and change are necessary, there is in the system as it is—both because of its strengths and despite its weaknesses—a wealth of medical experiences and raw life encounters to be had.

Most medical students hit the emotional skids more than once. At various times I have felt stupid, angry, frustrated, and nihilistic. Some of these feelings are inevitable at a time of transition; some are unique to the traumas of medical school: information overload, social contraction, first encounters with the body and with death. Some are generated by the failings of the school. But through all the disappointment, seeming futility, and personal problems, it is important to hold to the idea that you are engaged in an important and even profound process. Entwined within the jungle of anatomy, buried under the pyramids of pharmacology lists, and hidden in the maze of pathophysiology are some facts that actually help people. And behind the demands and disorientation of the clinical clerkships are not only chances to learn how medical science is applied, but opportunities to bring comfort and hope to sick people.

Perhaps I am getting carried away by idealism. Well, I wish idealism was a bit thicker around Harvard Medical School. It would have been a shot in an arm that was tired from lugging around big notebooks full of tiny facts. It would have given a more palpable purpose to the rote learning and ennobled the all-nighters on the wards. Idealism and inspiration are better than a cup of coffee when you are short on sleep. And, far from being antithetical to the science of medicine, they give it a meaning and context that make it more easily learned and humanely applied.

I hope others find more in medical school than is promised by the school catalog. They must not let themselves be blinded to the beauty and the sadness. There are exceptional models among the teachers here: the surgeon who makes house calls as well as elegant incisions; the cardiologist who is nearly as good at threading through the subconscious of his patients as he is at threading through their coronary arteries; the intern who has not become embittered; and the researcher who tries to capture students' curiosity with a question that has captured his for 25 years. Inspiration should be sought as diligently as clinical pearls. It comes in handy late at night. And its ultimate beneficiaries are patients.

Learning to be a doctor is necessarily hard. This does not mean that all of the hardship of medical school is necessary—but much of it is. While too much time is spent flaunting minutiae, there is no responsible way around learning a mind-bending amount of basic scientific and clinical material. And giving emotional succor to sick people under one's care is a more difficult task. However, to list only strains and stresses would be unfair as well as disheartening, for while the patients and doctors who have inspired me have not justified the faults or excessive demands of the school and the teaching hospitals, they have more than made up for them. In fact, inspiration has been provided often enough for me to consider it an essential part of medicine—perhaps the essential part.

Above all, these past few years have shown me medicine as a mixture of powerful contrasts: grief and joy, effectiveness and futility, humanity and callousness. It might appropriately be called a "mixed bag." Taking stock of its contents, examining them in light of these school years and pondering them against the glimmerings of the future, I cannot but conclude that it is a bag I want to keep.

Gringo-boy Comes Home to Practice Medicine: A Case Study of Professional Socialization at a Foreign Medical School

Robert H. Coombs

An estimated 12,000 to 15,000 U.S. citizens are currently enrolled in about 140 foreign medical schools, the majority of whom (75–90%) attend approximately ten schools in Mexico or the Caribbean. Yet, surprisingly, very little is known about the foreign experience. What little printed information exists typically deals with the performance of foreign trained doctors after they return to the United States. My three-year search located only one account of what life is like while studying medicine in a foreign country.[1] This is in marked contrast to the extensive literature about professional socialization in U.S. medical schools.[2]

To satisfy my own curiosity, I conducted lengthy tape-recorded interviews with two men (and one spouse) who had attended the same school in Latin America. One had just finished his second year, and the other, having completed all four years of foreign training, is now chief of a clinical service in a metropolitan hospital. Their experiences may or may not be typical of those trained at other schools. We won't know until other descriptions are published.

The case study that follows may be the first published account of the professional socialization experienced by medical students in a foreign land. To enhance readability, I have distilled and packaged verbatim commentary into a single account, the contents of which are both enlightening and provocative.[3]

My hope is that, in reading this narrative others will be stimulated to contrast their experiences, and that systematic research will be undertaken. Then prospective candidates for foreign *medical schools can have more realistic expectations of what awaits them.*

* * *

THE DECISION TO GO FOREIGN

I already had one mark against me; I could see the writing on the wall. After two years of applying and taking the MCAT, I was already about thirty years old. At most places, as soon as they saw my age, they said, "Sorry, you can no longer get into an American school; by the time you finish school, you'll not have enough years to give back to the public what they have invested in you." So I said, "O.K., fine!" and I packed to go foreign.

I realized, of course, that foreign medical training is not the optimum situation, but it was the only means available to me. The possibility of another career was deplorable to me. I was not ready to accept defeat. I was determined to make it, one way or another!

So I began investigating foreign settings. I spoke with people who had been in schools in the Philippines, in India, on the continent of Europe, in Mexico and the Caribbean, and other Latin American countries. There is not a great deal written about any of them. I wrote letters and they sent the standard brochures, noting the merits of their particular institutions. I considered them all. The whole world was open to me.

The idea of having to learn a new language did not traumatize me in the least. On the contrary, I looked forward to becoming fluent in a foreign language. And, partly because Ellen and I both love and have an affinity for the Spanish culture and language, we decided to go to Latin America.

Going out of the country seemed more of an adventure than a defeat. The idea of living in a foreign land, of getting to know the people and their customs intrigued us. So, the fact that people in our own land deemed me unacceptable was viewed as a temporary setback.

We ventured off as tourists to visit the school for three or four days and found the city to be charming, entertaining. The school looked good, too. They had whitewashed the buildings and they looked great. We met with some people who spoke fluent English whose job it was to sell the school. They welcomed us with open arms and encouraged us to make a formal application. We were very naive.

GETTING IN

I quickly learned that medical education at this school is a money-making operation. It's BIG, BIG business. The families that own the school are extremely wealthy and powerful people in their own country and have extensive properties in the United States. And they are very willing to take your money!

First of all, there is a $1,000.00 inscription fee that essentially buys you an interview. You hand it over to them and it goes right into the pockets of the owners of the university and makes them richer.

North American students were required to pay much more than Latinos. Natives paid for the entire four years what an American would have to pay for one semester. I calculated once that tuition cost North American students about $4 million per year, worth twice that amount in local currency. With all that money pouring in, they could have made it a quality medical school, but as far as I could see they never put one penny back into the system.

They required extensive background information on me—my original high school diploma, transcripts from junior high, even elementary school. These records had to be notarized and certified by the consulate. This cost $125.00. I'm sure that the United States government doesn't have a dossier on me like they do. It's unbelievable. They even wanted to know about my grandparents.

They copied U.S. requirements for undergraduate courses; chemistry and calculus and that sort of thing had to be on your transcript, but I doubt if they ever looked at this information. They have these little secretaries in charge of your files who barely know how to spell their own names.

After compiling all these documents and paying my $1,000.00 inscription fee, I presented myself for review and once again faced the possibility of rejection. I agonized, "If they reject me after paying the $1,000.00 and jumping through all these hoops, what then?" Feelings of insecurity welled up in me and I started questioning my validity. What would I tell my friends if I wasn't even accepted here? But I didn't hear of anybody who wasn't accepted. I think the $1,000.00 buys your way in.

So now I was accepted and feeling good about my life. I had finally gotten in at *SOME* medical school. So I packed up my belongings, said goodbye to family and friends, and set out on a new life. Although Ellen and I had to give up good jobs, a beautiful apartment, and a lot of valuable possessions, it was worth it. Hey, we're going to medical school!

IDEALISM AND DISILLUSIONMENT

I had to pass a mandatory language requirement before I could begin my medical studies. So I left Ellen for 3½ months to complete intensive language training offered on the main campus of the university. It proved to be the best part of my foreign education. I cannot speak more highly of the instructors or educational experience.

At the end of the intensive language training most of my classmates couldn't wait to get back to the U.S. But I did just the opposite. Ellen joined me and we went further into the interior, exploring the small pueblos and talking with the people. Getting a feel for the culture was fantastic.

Gung-ho from these experiences, we were surprised when American medical students warned us, "You don't have an accurate appraisal; you're in for a big surprise when you get to the medical campus." When I disputed them they said, "We'll see what you think a couple of months from now."

I vividly recall my first day of medical school. This was the day I had looked forward to for many years. I was a medical student at long last. I had shaved extra close, had my hair trimmed, and put on a tie and a pressed shirt. Today I was going to hear my first formal lecture in a medical setting—not as an observer but as a participant—and with tears welled up in my eyes I said to Ellen, "You, of all people, know how much this day means to me. I sincerely thank you for helping me and supporting me all this time to get where we are now."

Within three weeks my impression changed 180 degrees!

First of all, the facilities were nowhere near what they were purported to be. From the brochure, everything looked fantastic—nice new buildings fit for a picture postcard, with people surrounded by medical equipment (that they apparently commandeered for photographs). But you look inside and they are *nowhere* to be found. It's all a whitewashed facade—and I fell for it, hook, line, and sinker.

Our first class, histology, was held in a concrete room like a cell block. We called it "the catacombs" down there. Because it was bitterly cold there, I had to wear a sweater and a down vest to stay warm.

Cadavers were kept in huge vats tossed around with meat hooks by guys in big fishing waders. We called them "the goon squad." One day I walked by and saw one guy throwing out fetuses onto a tiled floor and then sweeping them into a big heap with a big barn broom.

Rather than having one cadaver for the entire semester as I had expected, we shared a cadaver with a large number of people on a session-by-session basis. In the morning five or six of us would use it, and at mid-day and then again in the evening other groups would be assigned to it. Then we'd see it again in two or three days.

The cadaver was in an advanced stage of deterioration and it was totally eviscerated. We never saw any organs at all, only bones and muscles that were almost impossible to delineate. To solve the cadaver shortage, some of my classmates actually bought bodies from a grave robber. When a friend told me of this I said, "You're pulling my leg." But it's the truth. Some squirrelly little gnome of a guy actually exhumes bodies from the cemetery at various stages of decay, and sells them to medical students. I wouldn't believe it if I hadn't seen it with my own eyes. It's like a horror film.

Classes began at 7.00 a.m. and they kept us there sometimes until 6:00 in the evening. They used up your whole day without teaching anything. I'd come home at 6:00 p.m. tired and livid with rage. It was audacious that they could waste so much time and subject us to all this busy work! It was emotionally draining.

The main goal of every single American I knew was to study your butt off for the boards and be able to transfer out. If you could do it this was the optimum situation.

Their main goal, by contrast, was not to educate us, but to keep us there for the duration of our medical education. For financial reasons they wanted us to stay, not transfer out. So they used up our time in class and busy-work assignments that had nothing to do with learning medicine. In this way they could dash any hope of transferring back into the U.S. as third-year students.

We were rarely educated by professors. Most of our class time was conducted by "pasantes," student teachers who were generally inept and extremely authoritarian. They loved to make us jump through time-consuming hoops, such as little homework assignments and preparing ridiculous write-ups. Class attendance was mandatory. Each of us had an assigned seat and every single day, without exception, they read off the attendance list. With 150 or more students per class, this would sometimes take half of the class time. They'd read off your number and you had to raise your hand and say, "Presente."

After we figured out that they weren't actually teaching us anything, only using up our time, every scam in the world was invented to try and get out of going to class. They countered by having guards walk up and down the aisles to make sure that you couldn't shift seats to answer to a friend's number.

Punishment resulted when too many classes were missed. Because they knew all the Yanks wanted to go home for Christmas, Spring break, and other holidays, those who missed class were required to pay a fine, take a more difficult second exam a week after the others had left, and receive, at best, a "C" grade. This "secundo vueltos" (second turn) policy forced us to choose between class attendance and going home.

Some of the teachers were openly anti-American. The only reason they tolerated us was for our money. They belittled us and browbeat us at every opportunity. Some, of course, were worse than others. The hostility of one guy was particularly distressing. He'd ask unanswerable questions and make a mockery of our inability to answer or speak the language, "What's the matter, American boy, you don't know the answer? You can't speak Spanish?"

SURVIVAL OPTIONS

Fighting back is not a viable option if one wants to eventually become a doctor. Either you leave or else you swallow your pride and play the game by their rules. They have the upper hand.

If you create trouble they retaliate by losing your grades, and then you have to repeat the entire semester. They lost my academic file three times while I was there; they had no record that I had ever been there and they made no effort to help me. The guy who I was supposed to see about my lost grades was unavailable and when I finally found him he insulted me and told me under no uncertain circumstances that he would not lift a finger to look for my records. He demanded that I sit for a second examination or I would be dealt with severely.

When I started to speak out, to complain, I was black-balled in two courses—biochemistry and physiology—and had to take the "segundo vueltos" and thereby forfeit my vacation. They said I had missed too many classes, but that was not true.

Amazingly, they even had an informant system. A select group of students, called "tecolotes" (owls), was employed by the medical school to watch for subversive activity. They were paid by the school to inform on those who would grumble or make objections. Although we hated the school and felt like airing our grievances, we had to be careful who we spoke to. I didn't know who among my Latin colleagues they were.

A few students left the school for moral reasons. Because of personal pride and integrity, they could not tolerate being party to humiliation and bribery. They felt prostituted when having to make concessions and pay sums of money in order to survive.

Those who stayed and survived, adopted the philosophy "play the game, pay the money, and you'll be a doctor in the end."

In this setting, you find out quickly that everything can be had for a price—including grades and special favors on examinations. Generally, if one is to survive, the system almost required that you "negotiate."

Sometimes students would get together and buy an exam. On one occasion the purchased exam was xeroxed and by the time we walked into the final exam almost every person had a copy. It was a farce.

Although there are exceptions most teachers are approachable. One said, "You be nice to me and I'll be nice to you." He made it clear that he liked gifts, and that if you were to complete the course you had better meet his expectations. It was almost a requirement. You were forced to participate, not just to improve your grade, but to insure that your grades wouldn't be lost.

One teacher was so blatant he would come up to you just before a final and say, "Look, you're going home for semester break, aren't you? This is what I want you to bring back if you want to pass this course." If you were unwilling to compromise your principles, you were in trouble. Even though you may have had a passing grade, they could either lose your grade or, if they wanted, retroactively change the grade and flunk you. That was their way of manipulating you. You were forced into playing their game.

If you're in academic trouble, no problem, you can buy your way out by approaching the teacher on a personal one-to-one basis and asking in a very open-ended way, "Is there any way that we can work this out?" Or if you are more bold, "Do you have any personal needs from the United States, like a TV set or stereo that would contribute to some teaching or research?"

When I took my first exams I was confident because I had studied hard and really had a handle on it. But when the results came back a couple of weeks later, I couldn't believe my eyes; I had not passed while Latino guys I knew didn't understand got high grades. Then, to make matters worse, the *pasante* called the gringos forward for a tongue lashing. "You're going to have to study much harder." I was livid with rage.

So what is the alternative if one is to survive? Take out an insurance policy—play the game by the local rules. This teacher loved to smoke very pungent cigars (at 7:00 a.m. in the lab!). So the day before the practical, my friend and I bought a $10.00 box of cigars and gave it to him to express our appreciation for all the "kindnesses" he had shown us during the semester. "Will you accept this gift as a small token of our appreciation?" we asked. All our friends had bottles of Johnny Walker Scotch or other little "presentos" for him.

You may not believe this, but during the exam this guy followed me around the lab from station to station whispering the correct answers in my ear. As I was focusing the microscope at one station, I heard "pssst." I looked up and there he was, whispering the answer. When he thought I did not understand, he gestured to help me understand the correct answer. I couldn't believe it. I sat back, then buried my head on my desk, biting my lower lip because I was laughing in disbelief. What would the folks back home think if they could only see me now?

SAFETY AND WELL BEING

There is an element of danger with you all the time. In order to become a doctor you risk not only your time, energy, finances, and emotions, you also risk you life!

Before I left for medical school, a friend encouraged me to buy a gun. When I protested that this was a ridiculous idea he said, "Let me urge you to carry a weapon; it's like an insurance policy. You may not have to use it, but if you do, you'll have it."

Although it's against the law for civilians to own weapons in this country, most people who can afford them own guns for self-protection. Although the biggest threat may come from hoodlums on the streets, the school itself is also an intimidating environment. It has its own armed police force and even professors sometimes carry weapons into class.

Let me tell you about our medical ethics professor (at least he led us to believe he was a professor). He started off the class with an offensive statement: "Classroom requirements are these: no sleeping, no talking, and no reading of pornography." Then he proceeded with a flamboyant presentation on the history of medical ethics. While writing high on the blackboard, he got his coat caught on the trigger guard of a revolver in a back holster and it flipped out onto the platform. Sweeping down like Errol Flynn, he picked it up, swept back his coat, and replaced the weapon, saying "disculpe" (excuse me). Then he proceeded with his lecture as though nothing had happened. I wondered, "Why would he feel the need to be armed in the classroom with a group of students?"

I later learned that guys like this carry weapons because, having been so abusive to American students, they fear for their lives. One guy in particular was loathed because he did everything to torment us. Not only did he lose our grades and require second exams, he called us "Gringo boys" and publicly ridiculed and belittled us. I've been told that on at least two occasions students departing the country had violently attacked him—once by a physical beating and another time by riddling his car with bullets.

Violence erupts in other ways, too. Murder is not uncommon and sometimes these came uncomfortably close to us at the medical school. Political hostilities are everpresent (such as that between the medical school and the nearby state school or with other Latin American countries). One political activist from a rival country, who had been kicked out of school, was denied medical care at the medical school clinic after he had sustained massive internal injuries by falling off a cliff while hiking. I knew him personally; a real sweetheart of a guy. They had told him, "Look, we don't want you making a lot of problems within your country's student population." He didn't meet their demands and ultimately died for it.

Every time I returned to school from my home in the United States, my guts would turn over. I was leaving all my personal freedom and rights that our constitution guarantees and preparing for combat. That's how I looked at it—to do battle according to their rules. I was entering a combat zone.

Near constant fear, humiliation, and rage take a toll on mental health. I noticed that a number of those approaching the end of their schooling seemed unusually distressed, even unstable. Even now when I get together with former classmates, I notice that they are still paranoid to some degree—glancing over their shoulders and talking out of the sides of their mouths when discussing the school. It's really pathetic.

RETURNING WITH STIGMA

My hat is off to each and every person who stayed in there and kept punching when they repeatedly got knocked down and abused. It takes a special breed to survive. They deserve commendation for their courage, their stamina, and their resourcefulness.

What hurts the most, though, is, having endured all this, to receive so much negative feedback about foreign-trained physicians. The pervasive attitude is that we aren't smart enough to get into a U.S. school, not qualified to be physicians, and will never be good doctors.

There is so much stigma attached to a foreign degree, some of my classmates who went the entire four years came to the U.S. and repeated the third and fourth years just so they could graduate with an American degree.

Most of us, though, go into a fifth pathway year. Because I wanted to be a really good doc I went into that year with a vengeance to learn. It was great to be back on good old U.S. terra firma. I knew that in one year I had to make up for two years of deficient clinical training. I also knew I had to take the Boards to get into a residency program and the Flex to be licensed.

Because of my deficiencies, there was a lot of pressure on me to prove myself, to excel. Besides taking care of ward duties, I had to spend a lot of time with the books learning a lot of things that others already knew. Some of the guys had a hard time handling that.

Some of the attendings expressed resentment towards us and regarded us as second-class medical students. When we couldn't answer a question they would cut us down, saying, "What's the matter? Didn't they ever teach you this in medical school? You should know this. You better get back to the books and learn this."

I remember numerous times when an attending would ask a question, and the U.S.-trained intern would come right back with the answer. Then the attending would turn and ask us another question and we couldn't answer. It just made us want to study harder.

During the fifth pathway year we acted as interns, being on call and doing a lot of the scutwork. But rather than being paid as other interns, we had to pay tuition for the privilege.

After this year of scutwork and intense study, I became a regular intern, a PGY-1. It was the same thing all over again, but this time I was getting paid for it and wasn't stigmatized. I was on equal grounds with the other interns and had made up for much of the deficiencies in my clinical training. At this point only a few people asked, "Where did you go to medical school?" They were more concerned with the quality of work that I could do. I didn't feel that I was labeled or had to prove myself any more than the others.

Getting into a good residency program was tough because most did not want foreign medical graduates. Even though I had completed a fifth pathway year, passed the Flex and all the rest, they still looked down on me. It was almost as if I had been blackballed by some specialties. But after I had been accepted, I was treated no differently than anyone else.

In private practice, the question of where I went to medical school hardly ever comes up. Other doctors want to know the type and quality of my residency training.

In some ways now I feel further ahead of my U.S.-trained colleagues. I can speak a foreign language, have been exposed to a lot more poverty, have familiarity with the nuances of the Latin culture and a great sensitivity to the needs of these people. About 20 percent of my patients now are Spanish-speaking.

I wouldn't have endured these experiences for any other purpose except medicine. I've lived to be not just a physician, but a *good* physician. I've realized my goal through struggle and hard work. I've surmounted all these obstacles. And it has been worth it.

ADVICE FOR THOSE WHO FOLLOW

My advice to pre-med students is, if you really want to be a doctor to the point that you can't shake it, have no alternatives, and can't get it out of your mind and heart, study like mad to get into a U.S. school!

If a foreign school proves to be your only alternative, be aware of the difficulties, frustrations and disappointments, and realize that there is no guarantee that you'll ever attain your goal. In the U.S. we have been raised on the American Dream—if you apply yourself, are honest and work hard enough, you can achieve anything you want. Through determination, resourcefulness, perseverance, and willingness to sacrifice you will eventually reach your goal.

That's a nice philosophy but it may not work if your goal is to become a doctor via a foreign medical school. From the day you arrive there will be formidable roadblocks, hurdles to overcome. You must have a gambler's spirit—to say, "I'll take all my money, my resources, my energy, years of my life, even risk my life, putting it on the line—and knowing full well that there are no guarantees."

But if you just can't get it out of your mind, wake up in the morning possessed with the idea of becoming a doctor and go to sleep dreaming about it—if you just can't shake it, then you've got to do it. Choose a school that teaches in English and prepares you for the Boards. And good luck. You'll need it!

NOTES

1. Carlos Pestana, *Foreign Medical Schools for U.S. Citizens*, San Antonio, 1983 (private publication, P.O. Box 32617, San Antonio, Texas 78216).
2. These books are among those that describe and analyze the experiences of students in U.S. Medical Schools: Becker, H. S., et al., *Boys in White*, University of Chicago Press, Chicago, 1963; Betcher, W. R., *A Student-to-Student Guide to Medical School: Study Strategies, Mnemonics, Personal Growth*, Little, Brown and Company, Boston, 1985; Bloom, S. W., *Power and Dissent in the Medical School*, The Free Press, New York, 1973; Broadhead, R. S., *The Private Lives and Professional Identity of Medical Students*, Transaction Books, New Brunswick, N.J., 1983; Coombs, R. H., *Mastering Medicine: Professional Socialization in Medical School*, The Free Press, New York, 1978; Coombs, R. H., and St. John, J., *Making It in Medical School*, Medicine and Society Press, Los Angeles, Peterson's Guides, Princeton, N.J., 1981; Coombs, R. H., and Vincent, C. E., *Psychosocial Aspects of Medical Training*, Charles C Thomas, Publisher, Springfield, Ill., 1971; Drake, D., *Medical School*, Rawson, Wade Publishers, Inc., New York, 1978; Fredericks, M. A., and Mundy, P., *The Making of a Physician*, Loyola University Press, Chicago, 1976; Gee, H. H., and Glaser, R. J., *The Ecology of the Medical Student: Report of the Fifth Teaching Institute Assn. American Medical Colleges, Atlantic City, New Jersey, October 15–19, 1957*, Evanston, Ill., 1958; Harrell, R. A., and Firestein, G. S., *The Effective Skut-boy*, Arco Publishing, Inc., New York, 1981; LeBaron, C., *Gentle Vengeance: An Account of the First Year at Harvard Medical School*, Richard Marek Publishers, New York, 1981; Martin, T., *How to Survive Medical School*, Holt, Rinehart and Winston, New York, 1983; Merton, R. K., et al., *The Student Physician*, Harvard University Press, Cambridge, 1957; Mullan, F., *White Coat, Clenched Fist*, MacMillan Publishing Company, Inc., New York, 1976; Shapiro, M., *Getting Doctored: Critical Reflections on Becoming a Physician*, Between the Lines, Ontario, Canada, 1978; Virshup, B., *Coping in Medical School*, Health Sciences Consortium, Inc., N.C., 1981.
3. Having published more than one-hundred manuscripts (including seven books), I was not unfamiliar with criticism, most of which has been instructive and helpful. But I was unprepared for the emotionally charged responses that this report stimulated. When an abbreviated version (less than 7 pages) was submitted to a medical journal for publication, 24 pages of criticism were returned. Apparently the manuscript had struck an exposed nerve with the reviewers. One completely rewrote my manuscript, inferring that I am incompetent. Others attacked the integrity of my sources, saying that there wasn't even a "hint of truth," only unsubstantiated rumors and gross exaggerations. One said, "It was a great, gross extrapolation to make these exaggerated, often ridiculous, and frequently incorrect comments when there are tens of thousands of such physicians who could be questioned in a coherent and logical fashion, and some real information, as opposed to disinformation, could be obtained." By contrast, another reviewer dismissed the findings as unremarkable: "Except for the mandatory language courses, the 'goon squad,' and 'graverobbers,' paid informants, and bribery of teachers, the dissatisfactions these men expressed, the busywork, long hours, required attendance, and playing the games (whatever the specifics may be) are common student complaints, whether foreign or U.S. Regarding weapons, I think any inter-city University hospital would have its share of 'armed citizens'—teachers and students included." Another reviewer felt that, although the report may accurately describe a less-than-ideal situation for U.S. students, it is implicitly a denunciation and therefore impolitic. "The reference to Latin America," he said, "would do nothing to bolster relations among the Americas."

RECOMMENDED READING

Premedical Education

Cook, Robert H., 1979, "The Narrow Gauge," *New England Journal of Medicine*, Vol. 301, No. 9, pp. 500–501.

Cookson, Clive, 1980, "Medical Schools Pressed to End Their 'Educational Birth Control,'" *New York Times* (Higher Education Supplement), Vol. 405, p. 4.

Coombs, Robert H., 1971, "The transition to medical school: Expectations versus realities," *Psychosocial Aspects of Medical Training*, R. H. Coombs and C. E. Vincent (eds.), Springfield, Ill., Charles C Thomas, Chap. 3, pp. 91–109.

Crovitz, Elaine, 1980, "Women Entering Medical School: The Challenge Continues," *Journal of American Medical Women's Association*, Vol. 35, No. 12, pp. 291–297.

Harvard Medical Alumni Bulletin, 1981, Special Issue or "The Premed Syndrome," Fall Issue, Vol. 55, No. 4.

Kielisch, Kurt D., 1984, "The MCAT Experience," *Pre-Med Advisor Magazine*, March Issue, pp. 5–6.

Nelson, Bernard W., 1981, "Liberal Arts and Humanities in Medicines," *The Pharos*, Fall Issue, p. 36.

Pestana, Carlos, 1983, *The Medical School Applicant: Advice for Premedical Students*, private publication, P.O. Box 32617, San Antonio, Texas 78216, 204 pp.

Powers, Robert D., 1984, "The MCAT Revisited," *The New England Journal of Medicine*, Vol. 310, No. 6, pp. 398–401.

Rose, John C., 1980, "The Admission Interview—Doing It to the Applicant," *The Pharos*, Summer Issue, pp. 13–14.

Wolf, Stewart G., 1978, "I Can't Afford a 'B,'" *The New England Journal of Medicine*, Vol. 299, No. 17, pp. 949–950.

Medical School

Altman, Lawrence K., 1982, "The Stresses of Medical School: A Smile Helps," *Harvard Medical Alumni Bulletin*, Vol. 56, No. 1, pp. 25, 60.

Anbar, Ran D., 1984, "Lessons from a Death," *The New Physician*, Vol. 33, No. 4, pp. 28–29.

Black, David, 1982, "The Making of A Doctor," *New York Times Magazine*, May Issues: May 23, pp. 18–26, 52–63, 75; May 30, pp. 20–28, 32, 35–39, 48.

Coombs, Robert H., *Mastering Medicine: Professional Socialization in Medical School*, The Free Press, New York, 1978.

Coombs, Robert H., and St. John, Joanne, 1981, *Making It in Medical School*, Medicine and Society Press, Los Angeles, California/ Peterson's Guides, Princeton, New Jersey.

Eisenberg, Carola, 1981, "Similarities and Differences between Men and Women as Students," *Journal of The American Medical Women's Association*, Vol. 36, No. 2, pp. 45–50.

Fink, Daniel J., 1971, "The First Year: Trial by Fire," *Journal of Medical Education*, Vol. 47, pp. 670–672.

Gibbs, Gladys Marie, 1981, "The Doctrine," *Harvard Medical Alumni Bulletin*, Vol. 55, No. 3, pp. 53–54.

Guggenheim, Frederick G., 1983, "On Clinical Clerkships: A Satirical Set of Rules," *The Pharos*, Winter Issue, Vol. 46, pp. 35–37.

Hoffman, Stephen, 1981, "Introduction to Ethical Medicine: A Student Examines Life on the Wards," *Harvard Medical Alumni Bulletin*, Vol. 55, No. 1, pp. 15–19.

Jason, Hilliard, and Westberg, Jane, 1979, "Toward a Rational Grading Policy," *New England Journal of Medicine*, Vol. 301, No. 11, pp. 607–610.

Larue, Annie, 1983, "Married to Medicine," *The New Physician*, No. 7, pp. 33–34.

Lief, Harold I., 1971, "Personality Characteristics of Medical Students," *Psychosocial Aspects of Medical Training*, Robert H. Coombs and Clark E. Vincent (eds.), Charles C Thomas, Springfield, Illinois, pp. 60–69.

Pestana, Carlos, 1983, *Foreign Medical Schools for U.S. Citizens*, private publication, P.O. Box 32617, San Antonio, Texas 78216, 176 pp.

Ringel, Marc, 1984, "Everyone Passes," *Pre-Med Advisor*, Summer Issue, p. 28.

Robinson, David Owen, 1978, "The Medical-Student Spouse Syndrome: Grief Reactions to The Clinical Years," *American Journal of Psychiatry*, Vol. 135, No. 8, pp. 972–974.

Rogers, David E., 1982, "Some Musings on Medical Education," *The Pharos*, Spring Issue, pp. 11–14.

Rosenberg, Donna A., and Silver, Henry K., 1984, "Medical Student Abuse: An Unnecessary and Preventable Cause of Stress," *Journal of The American Medical Association*, Vol. 25, No. 6, pp. 739–742.

Sacks, Michael H., Parker, Lynda, Kesselman, Martin, and Frosch, William A., 1980, "Psychiatric Problems in Third-Year Medical Students," *American Journal of Psychiatry*, Vol. 137, No. 7, pp. 822–824.

Silver, Henry K., 1982, "Medical Students and Medical School," *Journal of The American Medical Association*, Vol. 247, No. 3, pp. 309–310.

Stanley, Samuel L., 1981, "Last Night On," *Harvard Medical Alumni Bulletin*, Vol. 55, No. 1, pp. 29–31.

2

Postgraduate Medical Training: Internship, Residency, and Fellowship

Graduation from medical school is an achievement of great merit but is not recognized by practicing physicians as anything more than a beginning. Before one is acknowledged as clinically competent, additional years of intensive training must be successfully undertaken as a house officer—intern, resident, and perhaps fellow.

Historically, physicians at this stage actually resided in the hospital while working full time as an intern or resident. At Massachusetts General Hospital, one of our country's first and best-known teaching hospitals, the "Little Red House," where the original house physician resided, still exists on the grounds. These original residents received no salary, only board and room. In return, they were permitted to take care of patients as apprentices to the attending physicians.

Times have changed considerably since then. Housestaff receive salaries and no longer reside in the hospital, though there are notable exceptions, such as the trauma-team rotation at San Francisco General Hospital whose Chief Resident actually lives in the hospital for a month's period. Although less of an internment than originally, current residencies still remain highly confining. Today's housestaff maintain private residences, but most of their time is still spent in the hospital, especially when "on-call." Because these schedules may require work shifts of 36 hours or more, sleep is a luxury.

The length of time required to complete residency training varies from two to seven years or more, depending on the specialty. During the first year, referred to as Post Graduate Year 1 (PGY-1) all graduates must first complete an internship in internal medicine, surgery, or pediatrics. Afterwards, during PGY-2 etc., they become more deeply involved in specialty training. Anesthesia residencies require two years, while many surgical residencies take seven. The majority of other specialties, such as internal medicine, are somewhere between these extremes. Additional subspecialty training, called Fellowships, can extend the training period for an additional one to four years.

How are residencies arranged? Between September and December of their final year of medical school, soon-to-be physicians attire themselves in their most professional-looking garb and travel near and far to be interviewed by directors of residency programs. The outcome will not only determine how they begin their careers, but in what city they will live and who will be their friends and associates. The relative prestige of the teaching hospital will also, to some degree, confer professional success and self-worth.

Preceding these interviews, letters of recommendation from the medical school dean are mailed to appropriate residency program directors. With future careers at stake, as well as self-esteem, students naturally agonize about the contents of their letters and how well they will impress prospective employers.

Anxiety peaks in mid-March, when results of "The Match" are publicly announced. On this fateful day, classmates crowd into pre-arranged sites surrounded by wives, husbands, and babies who share in the excitement. Nervous tension is manifested by noisy chatter and uneasy joking. Cameras flash to preserve the memory. Then at noon the Dean hands out the envelopes and thousands of students from every part of the United States open them with exultant shouts or groans and tears of joy or frustration.

A computer in Evanston, Illinois, run by the National Residency Matching Program (NRMP), has matched student preferences of potential training programs (ranked from most to least preferred) with similar rankings of applicants by residency program directors and come up with the best possibility for each. But since student applicants typically outnumber the available positions, each year some students are publicly embarrassed.

Once settled into their new environment, newly minted physicians begin their internship. According to a dictionary definition, an intern is an inmate, one confined or detained within the limits of a specified place. This is an apt description of the medical internship, for much of this year passes within the confines of the hospital.

Of all the stages of professional development, the internship represents the physician's most significant rite of passage. At this time one becomes not only an M.D. (graduate of medical school), but also a "R.D." (real doctor). Medical school has taught the language, the basic vocabulary and syntax necessary to perform as an orthodox physician, but now the weight of personal responsibility for patient care is keenly felt. The young physician must now confront and deal with the constantly changing, frustrating, and uncertain world of hospital life. It is at this stage of training that personal gains in clinical skills and deficits in personal lifestyle are most strikingly apparent.

Work schedules of 90 to 120 a week often leave interns feeling physically and emotionally exhausted. Reflecting on his own internship, Casscells (1982) described his experience as "a blur." Because of the strenuous work days and the "conspiracy of silence," he says, interns feel isolated. There is little time to digest new information or communicate with others who are experiencing the same challenges. So each intern must weather the experience alone, without knowing if he or she is doing better or worse than others.

The typical intern works every weekday and spends every third night on duty in the hospital admitting new patients and handling emergencies. This means that the intern must work a hectic 36-hour shift at least twice a week. On a bad night, sleep may consist of only 2 or 3 hours.

If the intern's income, typically about $20,000 per year, is divided by hours worked, the hourly wage approximates the minimum wage.

The intense pressures felt during this time are vividly portrayed by this intern:

> I remember a friend two or three years ahead of me saying, "Now Susan, it's going to get tough. When you get upset, just go into the bathroom and cry your heart out and you'll feel better." I said, "What? I don't cry! I never cry! I'm tough! I can take it!" But unless you've been under the stress of an intern or house officer you'll never know. Unless you've had the experience of doing all the scutwork, standing up under the pressure of criticism for failure to perform like Hercules, you'll never know.
>
> I can remember one of my most horrendous nights on call, when I had spent all my time in the intensive care unit working on this man who was obviously going to die, and I thought it was a sin that he should have to submit to all these things that we were doing to him. Even though I thought it totally unethical, I had to do these procedures because of my orders. There was no way I could not, as I was new, and I didn't know enough to be able to say, "No, I won't do that."

So all through the night I agonized. I spent the entire night in the unit with him. To make matters worse I had four admissions that night, three of whom required close supervision, and I couldn't give it to them. I had to do all the lab work—the blood cultures, and the sputums, and everything else. I was going nuts!

By the end of the night, about 6 o'clock in the morning, the first guy died. It was a hopeless case. When I finally got back to one of my other patients, I found him going down the tube because of pneumonia. I hadn't been able to watch him carefully. Then, during 8 o'clock rounds, I was asked about my four patients, and I couldn't remember who was Mr. Smith and who was Mr. Brown; they all looked the same. The chief resident, a really tough, very secure, very bright guy who gets real hard-nosed, drilled me and said, "You don't know what happened last night, do you?"

Then I started screaming at him. "You're damned right I don't know what's going on," I said. "I spent all night long in the intensive care unit and had four admissions, none of which I was adequately able to work up, although I did what was necessary. They're all on their antibiotics, other medications—but you're right, I don't remember who has what at this moment." Then I knew I was going to cry, so I walked down the hall, went into a bathroom, and cried my eyes out.

Many of the trials and tribulations of the intern year apply as well to subsequent years of residency training, but usually the stress is not as great. The time demands are somewhat reduced and the actual direct responsibility for patient care slightly less strenuous. But new stressors, as well as new sources of satisfaction, are added. For one thing, residents (PGY-2 and beyond) are more accountable than interns for the ultimate progress of patients, so that the "buck" tends to stop with them. Residents also do more teaching than interns; they supervise both the medical students and the interns in their clinical work. For some residents, teaching is challenging and exciting, but for those who doubt their own professional competence, teaching can be a frightening responsibility.

As one observer noted (Hunter, 1976) residents wear many "hats." Among them are (1) employee of the hospital, (2) clinician, a licensed professional caring for sick patients, (3) post-doctoral student, (4) the teacher of medical students, junior physicians, and other health personnel, (5) administrator of a complex health team, and (6) participating investigator involved in clinical research.

Because these roles are typically carried out in urban teaching hospitals, described by Hunter (1976) as one of the most complicated social institutions ever to evolve, the resident's experience can be "an administrative nightmare." "There, in the midst of a biologic revolution and a revolution in health-care expectations on the part of the public," Hunter says, "life-and-death decisions are being made around the clock, 365 days a year, Christmas and the Fourth of July included." Is it any wonder that young residents sometimes feel overwhelmed and bewildered.

When, in order to find relief, residents occasionally leave the familiar hospital corridors for a change of scenery and some fresh air, ever-present beepers may beckon them back. Although these electronic gadgets enhance communication, they add to the frenzy of a resident's life, as this comment from a neurology resident illustrates:

> The most stressful part of my work on a day-to-day basis has to do with people wanting me to be at three, four, and sometimes five places at precisely the same time, and all these demands of equal legitimacy. It's very, very stressful!
>
> I just hate to be in the middle of working up a patient in the emergency room and just about ready to listen to the heart or whatever, and the beeper goes off and I have to trot out to the nearest phone to find out what's wanted. Since there isn't a phone nearby (this isn't a very classy hospital), I have to traipse down the hall to the closest telephone.
>
> And just as you're thinking you might be able to figure out what's wrong with the poor guy in the emergency room, there's someone in the ICU who also needs your immediate attention. And then, as you're walking back down the hall to the emergency room, the beeper goes off again! It's very stressful to hear. Three or four different interns may need a neurology consult now, and you need to respond. It's hard to remain unruffled inwardly, as well as outwardly, when constantly interrupted.
>
> After a while, you learn that the intern or resident who's calling you is probably over-reacting a little. You learn that when some people see a seizure they panic, though to you it's not serious. Surgeons especially will do that. You hear anxiety in their voice, and though you realize it's not a life-threatening situation, you can't tell them, "I'll be there in half an hour." You have to explain to them that it is not really an emergency. You can't say, "Ah, you jerk, that's not an emergency." You say instead, "I think the situation is under control. There are a couple of other things you could do 'til I get there. Do this, this, and that; I think you're doing a good job. I'll be there in thirty minutes." In general, a calm, kind voice reassures hospital people who are very uptight. It relieves their panic and it helps them know that things are OK, that not everybody's going to die here tonight.

But sometimes *I'm* panicking in my heart when I'm called five places at once. But I try not to let anybody see that, because it just adds to their anxieties.

At the completion of residency training, additional specialized training as a Fellow can be taken in any one of a number of subspecialties such as cardiac surgery, child psychiatry, endocrinological gynecology, or ultrasound radiology. Internal medicine alone offers a variety of subspecialty training opportunities, a few of which are gastroenterology, hematology, cardiology, and rheumatology. Varying from one to four years, this training provides in-depth experience in a narrowly specialized realm of practice.

The motivations for doing a fellowship are varied: feeling a need for more in-depth training, wanting to delineate a more narrow area of clinical responsibility, not feeling ready for independent private practice, wanting to develop an academic track, or wanting to enhance income or prestige. Because of increasing technological developments and competition for patients, an increasing proportion of residents elect to do subspecialty fellowships thus influencing the course of medical practice for many years to come.

Fellows earn roughly the same income as residents, but they typically supplement their income by moonlighting, working at a second job after hours and on days off; but, in general, they are not free to set up a private practice. During this time, fellows may remain under the control of the Department Chairperson and subject to the policies that regulate all house officers. In some highly competitive fellowships like cardiac surgery, ones that ensure a lucrative private practice, no salary may be offered at all.

The lifestyle of a fellow is typically more relaxed than that of an intern or resident. As a resident he or she may have worked 60–90 hours a week, but as a fellow the work week is now closer to 40–70 hours. One reason is that, in most fellowships, admitting patients is no longer a responsibility. A pediatric surgical fellow, on a beeper at home, for example, comes to the hospital when either the pediatric or surgical resident determines that a child needs acute surgical attention. However, many fellowship programs still require great amounts of clinical work from their fellows, particularly in tertiary care centers that deal with complicated clinical diseases, or when the department chairperson lacks confidence in the residents.

What happens when house officers become sick? Frequently pushing themselves beyond the limits of strength and endurance, and constantly exposed to contagious organisms, residents may succumb to illness. This can be depressing for anyone, but imagine the psychic conflict created within a young physician trained to maintain control in the face of exhaustion, fear, and uncertainty and dedicated to beating disease. To publicly surrender to illness, letting oneself be treated as a patient, is for them an admission of defeat. The personality qualities which have helped them appear success- ful—intellectualizing, control, and mastery—are counterproductive when experiencing personal illness. Because the sick role with its requisite traits—acceptance, passivity, and dependence—requires the opposite of that expected of physicians, these qualities may be used as a defense mechanism when the physician becomes ill. When combined with alcohol or other drugs, denial can have self-defeating results. But, for many physicians, the alternative (patienthood) is worse.

These and related topics are explored in the articles that follow.

The first selection, "The Chief," written by an anonymous intern, provides a portrayal of an intern's day on a busy medical ward. The interpersonal networks in the pressured environment of the teaching hospital are colorfully described. The principle charac- ters in this account are: (1) the kindly Chief, an intellectually intense physician who arises between four and five in the morning to help his teenage son with his homework and then at 5:30 a.m. delivers a lecture to the resident staff, (2) the highly critical and demanding research-oriented attending physician, who is more eager to compile data than to help patients, and (3) the surgery resident who, when called for a consult, remarked, "a chance to cut is a chance to cure." This slice-of-life view captures a feeling of what it is like when struggling to stay one step ahead of death and keep out of trouble with demanding mentors and other associates.

The second selection is an editorial by Norman Cousins, who asks a volatile question—is the internship experience preparation or hazing? In Cousins' view, the internship is the weakest link in the chain of physician training. Much like a "human meatgrinder," he says, it is "disguised hazing at best and systematic desensitization at worst," a process not only detrimental to newly minted physicians but also to their patients. What kind of judgement, he asks, can be expected from a physician who hasn't slept in 32 hours?

The response elicited by Cousins' editorial illustrates the intensity of feelings that most physicians have about this subject and provides a good overview of contrasting views. According to the journal editor, an "avalanche" of thoughtful commentary came in response. Of the 22 that were printed as representative, 6 agree with

Cousins and 16 disagree. Most of the latter, written with considerable intensity, point out that the pressure has a purpose. The internship, they say, is a period of great growth and accelerated learning, a time that solidifies the learning of medical school, and is crucial in the development of clinical judgement. They ask, how else can one learn whether he or she is capable of dealing with crisis?

"Stress During the Internship Year," by Joel E. Dimsdale, a professor of psychiatry at Harvard Medical School, presents results of personal interviews with twelve interns. Social and personal lifestyles are examined, as are physical and emotional well-being. Dimsdale concludes that, since the internship is such an extremely stressful period, considerable planning is needed to deal with stressors that may be counterproductive to the well-being of interns and the patients they serve.

"House Officer Stress Syndrome," by Gary W. Small, describes the anger, cynicism, and other responses which, in one form or another, affect nearly every house officer. House officers (i.e., interns and residents) face many stresses, such as sleep deprivation, excessive workload, patient care responsibility, fear of fatal errors, constantly changing work conditions involving frequent rotations to new floors and wards, and peer competition that may lead to social isolation. "The house officer stress syndrome" that may follow from these conditions has seven characteristics: (1) episodic cognitive impairment (mostly due to sleep deprivation), (2) chronic anger and resentment, (3) pervasive cynicism, (4) family discord, (5) depression, (6) suicidal thoughts and actions, and (7) alcohol and drug abuse.

The author points out, however, that residency stress is not all bad since it may enhance clinical competence. In order to promote the advantageous aspects of residency training while reducing the detrimental features, Small suggests a number of practical changes, such as reducing the work hours, providing support groups, and, if necessary, psychiatric referrals.

The next selection, "The Goal," written by an anonymous spouse of a sixth-year surgical resident, provides a glimpse of how a prolonged residency can impact on marriage and family life, a relatively unexplored topic. This poignant account documents, in a step-wise fashion, the ebbing of life from the resident's family as more and more of his life is dedicated to surgical training. It is a familiar but sad revelation of how a young physician, described by his wife as a humanitarian, can win the battle (achieve "The Goal") while losing the war (his family). "We made it through medical school and most of residency," his wife points out. "We coped for a long time, in our different ways." Then she sorrowfully adds, "His patients should be grateful. Their bright young surgeon has been skillfully trained but selfishly possessed by a system that forgets that behind many good residents are their families, waiting."

Suzanne Trupin's article, "When the Obstetrician Gets Pregnant," is the story of what happens when a Chief Resident in Obstetrics and Gynecology becomes an expectant mother. If medical center folklore is correct that doctors are the worst patients, then resident obstetricians, she asserts, are "the worst of the worst." For one thing, the possession of medical knowledge may stimulate fears. A physician is more acutely aware of all that can go wrong and of the various risks, such as infection, difficult deliveries, and the possibility of a damaged or stillborn baby.

The decision to have a baby at this busy time brought "flack" from the program director and residents. So, realizing full well that her colleagues, other harried housestaff, must take on the additional burden of her work left undone, she did not take the time for herself that she would have advised for her patients.

When enrolled in a Lamaze course for expectant mothers, Trupin felt the need to conceal her identity as an Obstetrician. Being a medical expert and a patient don't fit. But despite these problems, she said, it was well worth the trouble for the rewards were great, not only in terms of motherhood, but also in professional growth. Her first-hand experience helped her become more emphatic and understanding of her pregnant patients. Being able to share personal experiences—as well as medical expertise—made her a more sensitive, understanding, and effective physician.

A less happy exposure to the patient role came to Scott May during his last year of a Child Psychiatry Fellowship. His interesting account, entitled "Overnight in the CCU," documents his 24-hour experience as a patient in the Coronary Care Unit of a busy university hospital. In this insightful narrative, the author discusses the effect that this role reversal, from physician to patient, had upon his thoughts and feelings. May's brief sojourn as a patient highlights the special assets and liabilities that may evolve when a physician is suddenly thrust into the sick role and forced to confront his own illness. Becoming a patient, he says, was not only a hassle, but "a blow to my dwindling sense of omnipotence. It was a real psychological crunch."

But there is an up-side to this, as May and Trupin each acknowledge. If a physician can successfully navigate the difficult transition from physician to patient and then back to physician, he or she may gain invaluable personal insights about patient experiences and thus become a more effective healer. The experience may help the physician descend from the icy slopes of Mount Olympus to the real world of daily practice where healing actually takes place.

REFERENCES

Casscells, W., 1982, "Life (so to Speak) after Medical School: The Method and Madness of Internship," *Harvard Alumni Bulletin*, Vol. 56, No. 1, pp. 22–24, 60. •
Thomas H. Hunter, 1976, "Sounding Board: How Many Hats Can A House Officer Wear?" *The New England Journal of Medicine*, Vol. 294, pp. 608–609.

The Chief

Anonymous

The chief did homework with his oldest son every morning between 4 and 5 a.m. They would work together on trigonometry or biology—whatever the son was studying in high school. It had to be that early because it was the only time the chief had available. By 5:15 a.m. he would be smoking his seventh or eighth cigarette and brewing his second pot of coffee of the morning. Then he would prepare his morning lecture for the medicine house staff that began at 5:30 a.m.

I was not the best or most dedicated intern, and I seldom came to the lectures more than three times a week. The talks usually concerned cardiology, which was the chief's specialty. I am not particularly interested in cardiology, but it never occurred to me at the time because when he explained an ECG or an angiogram, I became interested.

The chief was thin and wiry. He had an intellectual intensity that was infectious, but, more important, he had an unaffected kindness and concern that won your loyalty. On rounds, he would converse for hours with unkempt old men who had been admitted to the hospital with atypical chest pain. The chief would have all the house staff bobbing to and from the patient's chest with their stethoscopes; the patient would be jumping like a hooked trout from the left lateral decubitus position onto his back and then to the sitting position as we all listened to his heart. The chief cared about these patients and their chest pains, even though most of the rest of us were bored by the long, complicated histories.

Often, late in the evening, the chief would pop his head into a patient's room and find me at the bedside of an acutely ill patient; he was always glad to see me there.

"Clinical judgment comes from experience," he would say, and he would often be waiting at the nursing station to discuss the case when I finished with the patient. It was reassuring to discuss these cases with him, and even when he wasn't actually present during a crisis, it seemed like he was.

One afternoon the admitting resident called me about a new patient. He was Earl Swenson, a 73-year-old man with emphysema, arthritis, and (thanks to his recently prescribed arthritis medication) a bleeding ulcer.

"I've got a GI bleeder for you," he told me. "I don't think that he's bleeding much now, but you'd better come quick to collect him. The unit resident already turned him down. Not sick enough, I guess."

This was baleful information. No intern was happy about admitting a gastrointestinal bleeder at that time. The surgeons and the gastroenterologists were working on studies comparing the effectiveness of medical and surgical therapies for patients with bleeding ulcers. Since Mr. Swenson had been admitted to me, he would be treated medically. A gastroenterologist would soon arrive to assess my treatment of the patient. Meanwhile, I had to request the chief resident on surgery to see the patient in consultation.

When the surgeon arrived, he cheerfully suggested that I perform every diagnostic and therapeutic procedure that he could think of on the spur of the moment. He then intimated that by denying my patient the definitive, surgical therapy, I shared in the responsibility for any morbidity that might occur.

"A chance to cut is a chance to cure," he explained as he strode off.

Marvin Walters was the attending gastroenterologist who consulted on Mr. Swenson's case. He arrived hopping mad and eager to find fault.

"Why isn't this man in the intensive care unit?" he demanded.

"I guess the unit resident didn't think that he was having a serious enough hemorrhage," I answered.

"I'll talk with him later. As for you, you'd better not make any mistakes on the study protocol," he warned.

I realized as Walters stalked off that Mr. Swenson was important to him. Not only would he be another successful case in his study, but Swenson's example would be a valuable bludgeon to use against the surgeons and on the rheumatologists for having prescribed the medication that caused the ulcer.

Luckily, my other patients were stable, and I was able to spend the evening with Mr. Swenson and to talk with him and his daughter. I inserted a central venous pressure line, started a large-bore intravenous tube for transfusing blood, and carried out all of the procedures and tests required by the study. While Mr. Swenson underwent his stomach X-ray studies, I filled out all of the information in the gastroenterologists' study protocol chart.

As the evening progressed, there was little bleeding, but at about 1 a.m., the aspirate from Mr. Swenson's nasogastric tube turned bloody, his pulse rate speeded up, and his intestine began to churn. I tried various techniques to quell the bleeding, and I began to transfuse him with whole blood, but soon I could tell that I was simply keeping ahead of the bleeding. I watched, fascinated, as Mr. Swenson's physiological functions responded to my therapy and then drifted away again as the bleeding continued. There was no doubt that he needed to be transferred to the intensive care unit for selective pitressin therapy and for continued, close monitoring.

Mr. Swenson slept most of the time that I worked at his bedside over the next few hours. At about 4 a.m. I thought about the chief. He was probably working with his son. I realized that by his example the chief also had been trying to teach me something. Finally, during the night I realized that I was learning this important lesson. I felt exultant. I and I alone knew about the seriousness of Mr. Swenson's bleeding, and I knew from first-hand experience. Although the bleeding was rapid, I could keep him out of trouble. I knew what had to be done.

Soon, morning came, and right after our morning rounds I arranged to transfer Mr. Swenson to the intensive care unit. When I returned to his bedside I found Marvin Walters haranguing my resident. Mr. Swenson and his daughter cowered as Walters paraded around the bed.

"I warned that intern I wouldn't tolerate any mistakes," he said. "This patient should have been in the intensive care unit to begin with, and now this happens!" Then, noticing me, he called, "Get over here! How could you let this happen?"

"What's wrong?" I asked numbly. "Is Mr. Swenson's bleeding worse?"

"I don't care about bleeding," Walters yelled, "Nobody recorded the data in the study chart this morning. Now we can't use this patient in our study! You'll kill this old man yet!"

With these words, Walters and his students marched out of the room leaving me and my resident to pick up the pieces of our shattered relationship with the Swenson family and explain that, yes, Mr. Swenson would have to be treated in the intensive care unit, just like Dr. Walters said. Walters refused to listen when told that the data he wanted were sitting on a piece of paper at Mr. Swenson's side and that I just hadn't had a chance to transfer the information to the study chart. He refused to have anything more to do with the case.

As the resident went off to the usual morning report meeting with the chief, I sat staring at the wall in the intern's office, exhausted from lack of sleep and despondent about my dismal failure with Mr. Swenson. I have no idea how much later it was when the resident returned and informed me, "The chief wants to see you." Bathed in gloom, I walked to the chief's office. He greeted me as usual, and after we sat down in his office, he asked me how Mr. Swenson was doing. I immediately confessed my mistakes. I explained that Mr. Swenson should have been transferred to the intensive care unit earlier, but that I hadn't realized it until during the night when the bleeding intensified. Also, I told him, it had been my responsibility to transfer the monitoring data to the study chart. I had known that Dr. Walters was going to be seeing Mr. Swenson this morning. He had warned me not to make any mistakes on the protocol, but I had neglected to finish it on time.

"I'm afraid I let you down on this case," I told the chief, and my eyes stung.

The chief cleared his throat and said, "Well, of course, minor errors do occur, but I think that on the contrary, you have given Mr. Swenson excellent care. You were at his bedside the whole night. He couldn't have been watched more closely even in the intensive care unit. The reason I wanted to talk with you this morning was simply to tell you how proud I am of your effort for Mr. Swenson."

"Also," he confided in a quieter tone as we rose to walk to the door of his office, "I feel sure that Dr. Walters, when he is made aware of all of the details of the case, will want to apologize to you and to the Swenson family for his misleading remarks."

I wanted to say so much to the chief. To thank him, to apologize for the times that I had let him down, to tell him how much I respected him, but instead, all I could stammer was something about how maybe with experience I would develop clinical judgment.

I must have been walking a bit unsteadily because the chief put his arm on my shoulder as we walked back toward the ward.

"I have another homily that I reserve for occasions such as this," he told me. "Good judgment comes from experience, but unavoidably, experience comes from bad judgment."

We laughed at this paradox and he told me, "Get a nap. I'll see you at the noon seminar."

Internship: Preparation or Hazing?

Norman Cousins and Responding Physicians

INTERNSHIP:
PREPARATION OR HAZING?

For the past two years, I have been privileged to visit medical schools and hospitals in various parts of the country. I have been able to meet with medical students and physicians at various stages in their training and their careers. The weakest link in the entire chain of physician training, it seems to me, is the ordeal known as the internship. More specifically, I refer to the theory that it is necessary to put medical school graduates through a human meat grinder before they can qualify as full-fledged physicians. Putting it more delicately, the theory holds that anyone who wants to go into the medical profession must be given a rigorous and systematic exposure to the realities of the physician's life.

How does the internship prepare the physician for the "realities?" What if the "preparation" has the effect of dulling the sensitivities of the physician, or fostering feelings of resentment by an intern toward a patient who has a propensity for feeling his sharpest pains at 3 a.m.? What kind of judgment or scientific competence is it reasonable to expect of a physician who hasn't had any sleep for 32 hours? Is the workload at times not so much a sampling of later challenges as it is an exercise in what I can describe only as disguised hazing at best and systematic desensitization at worst? Is it a good policy to subject seriously ill patients to treatment by physicians who are physically and emotionally exhausted? It was interesting and significant to me that the defense of the practice came from those who, having survived the experience, seemed determined not to permit others to escape. For the most part, however, I found that most physicians, on or off hospital staffs, saw little justification for the practice and, indeed, expressed serious reservations about it.

Some of the most productive discussions I had about the institution of the internship were in the open forums accompanying the grand rounds to which I was invited by various hospitals. Not infrequently, the subject of physician–patient relationship would come up. It was recognized that the physician should take the initiative in this matter, to obtain the patient's full confidence as well as to promote confidence by the patient in his own healing system. Among the physician's useful attributes, it was generally agreed, was a supportive and compassionate attitude toward the patient.

It was at this point, however, that the discussion would break wide open. The physicians would generally say that the internship was hardly conducive to feelings of compassion toward patients. They pointed out that seeing patients under conditions of pressure and fatigue is no more satisfying for the physician than it is for the patient. One of the former interns would be certain to point out that having a man with a bloodstained knife come at you in the emergency room is enough to quiet the compassionate urgings in most doctors' souls. Another physician said he was ashamed to admit that he hoped (generally at 3 a.m.) that his call-button-pressing patient would die before he got there. Compassion, apparently, is favored by circumstance.

In general, the most frequent question that was raised concerned public responsibility. How did the practice of "round-the-clock" medicine affect the patients themselves? One of the interns said it was difficult for him to see how medical administrators could defend themselves against charges of poor judgment by physicians on prolonged duty. At a time when the public is malpractice-suit prone, it would appear that the vulnerability of the hospital, medical school, or both to legal action would be sufficient to change the custom.

Over and above these specific problems is a matter I mentioned a moment ago: to what extent do the burdens placed on the interns come more under the heading of hazing than conditioning? Is a harsh and punitive attitude by some residents toward interns an essential part of the training of young physicians? Is it possible that some residents enjoy and exploit their power over the newcomers? Does hazing of this sort reflect credit on the profession? Is it really necessary?

The custom of overworking interns has long since outlived its usefulness. It doesn't lead to the making of better physicians. It is inconsistent with the public interest. It is not really worthy of the tradition of medicine.

Norman Cousins
Program in Medicine, Law,
and Human Values
UCLA School of Medicine
Los Angeles

INTERNSHIP:
PHYSICIANS RESPOND TO NORMAN COUSINS

Editor's note: Following publication of Norman Cousins' article concerning internship (1981; 245:377), we received an avalanche of thoughtful commentary. We have selected excerpts from some of the correspondence and offer them here with Norman Cousins' response. I wish to thank Micky Forbes for preparing this column and Mr. Cousins for his kind cooperation.—L.D.G.

Norman Cousins has taken the rigors of internship to task, likening it to hazing, which serves no useful purpose. Having survived the institution with no ill effects, I believe he is wrong.

The purpose of internship is to make the transition from the sheltered lap of academia into the at times harsh world of real patients and disease. As an intern, one learns to apply the knowledge gained during medical school. Medicine differs fundamentally from other disciplines in that disease does not submit to an 8-to-5 routine. It occurs at unpredictable hours, and if one is to observe it at first hand, one must be there when it happens. To do this, there is no substitute for long hours and frequent night calls spent in the hospital. One must spend days and nights in the hospital not only to see disease when it arrives, but to follow up closely its course in patients.

When one becomes a physician, one assumes responsibility for patients. This is a seven-day-a-week, 24-hour-a-day commitment. There is no way to avoid it other than choosing a support specialty. This does not mean that one works all the time, but what it does mean is that one accepts the commitment to take care of one's patients when they become ill. A large part of internship resides in teaching this fundamental fact and conditioning the reflexes to act on it even when one is tired, ill, or lazy.

James D. Leitzell, M.D.

At the time I was an intern it seemed a cruel price to pay to become a "full-fledged physician." I could not understand why my resident insisted on reviewing the same things over and over again, why I had to respond continuously, sometimes for 72 hours in a row. What good could it possibly do me to see my fifth gastrointestinal bleed in the same day? What good could it possibly do me to put my third subclavian in within 40 minutes? What good could it possibly do me to recognize the difference between a migraine headache and a subarachnoid hemorrhage when surely time would tell anyway? In retrospect I found it to be one of the most rewarding experiences that I have ever been through.

L. J. Turkewitz, M.D.

I read with great appreciation Norman Cousins' essay, "Internship: Preparation or Hazing?" Any of us young enough to look back on internship days with clear lenses relives in memory the errors made when dropping from fatigue. At least two recent studies have demonstrated the naivete of assuming that interns are immune from the need for sleep. Who would willingly fly in a plane whose pilots had been awake for 36 hours? I've learned not to take umbrage at the lowly intern who nods during my rounds. A little imaginative planning would easily solve the problem, but first we must reshape a lot of attitudes.

Oscar D. Ratnoff, M.D.

I seriously doubt that Norman Cousins ever completed the internship he vilifies and thus his opinions strike me as worthless. He betrays his ignorance in picking 32 hours as an excessive length of time to work. That is just 8 a.m. until 4 p.m. the next day. He should have picked the more typical surgical call of 5 a.m. until 8 p.m. the next day.

Mr. Cousins assumes there is a direct correlation between how much sleep a man has and his compassion and judgment. Rather, these are more proportional to the person's temperament and character. In fact, the physicians to whom I would trust my care happen to be quite busy and "overworked."

Am I to assume we won World War II because we had more sleep? Would Henry Ford and Thomas Edison have not been great without their beauty sleep? On the contrary, I'm sure they put in many 24-, 36-, and 48-hour days. The tenor of Cousins' whole discussion is that of some bleeding heart from the Occupational Safety and Health Administration who underestimates human strength and the will to succeed. Small wonder mediocrity rules America!

Donald C. Faust, M.D.

Internship, the high-pressure, hell-of-a-hazing year that introduces most physicians to the real world of medicine outside medical school, deserves some praise. Lack of sleep has its benefits. In what other business could an 80-hour week be called "short"? How else could one learn the joys of sleeping in until 7 a.m. or getting three hours of uninterrupted sleep? In what other job would one be forced to make life or death decisions on less than an hour's sleep, let alone have no chance to "sleep on" a major decision?

Harsh as this sounds, the pressure has a purpose. Only in a semiprotected environment like internship can physicians learn whether or not they are capable of dealing with crises and, if not, change directions before wasting time in an unhappy situation.

Susan Reitz, M.D.

I wish to applaud Mr. Cousins' comments. I hope they will stimulate a reevaluation of the long hours required of interns and residents. It is time for the medical profession to realize that the problems of stress, sleep deprivation, and fatigue apply to physicians as well as patients. Government already regulates the flying hours of airline pilots in the interest of public safety. If physicians do not regulate themselves, government regulation may be the result.

Gary Shugar, M.D.

Pope wrote:

Drink deep, or taste not the
   Pierian spring:
There shallow draughts intoxicate
   the brain.

Mr. Cousins' information concerning the "ordeal of internship" and the putting of convenience above the lives of patients arises, I suspect, from a mixture of outlandish anecdotes and overly accented criticisms designed to shock the inquirer and amuse the teller.

Never did I or my fellow interns, who walked silent and compassionate through dark wards filled with the smell and rustle of suffering, ever wish for the quick death of any patient to relieve us of our duties. Never were we more alert and more capable, even after long wakeful hours, than when we struggled with the enemy, Death.

Frank Vogel, M.D.

I have worked in teaching hospitals many years and have seen the rigorous schedules interns are continually put through in the name of "educational experience." Because this is the way the physicians heading the programs had to learn, these new physicians are subjected to the same. One would hope that these "teaching" physicians would have remembered the difficulties imposed on them as a result of being up 32 hours on call after a full week of constant on-the-go schedule. How can a physician be expected to function and make coherent patient care decisions in a state of fatigue? Doesn't the patient who is now paying premium prices for hospital care deserve more? The medical profession must continually be aware of changes in methods of treatment and of the new drugs that become available. Why is it not also aware of the continual need to update and change the methods by which it is educated?

Barbara McInturff

During the last 30 years, a variety of circumstances have dramatically changed the fortunes of first-year medical postgraduates, no matter what their specialty. First of all, their pay scale is commensurate with their training and capability, and it allows them to live respectably, even if married. Second, the work load has dramatically diminished. Interns, in general, are not required to perform any laboratory work, with the possible exception of primary urinalyses and blood work under conditions of extreme emergency. And, last but not least, the custom of around-the-clock unending call has long since been discontinued, at least in the environs where I practice. Most house staff are released after evening rounds, leaving those persons on immediate call to cover the house and perform the workups on newly admitted patients. This is such a dependable and predictable situation that people in the first year of postgraduate training are reliably able to contract themselves as "moonlight" physicians in other hospitals.

Fred T. Caldwell, Jr, M.D.

Many physicians who complained of their internship later come back to look at it as the time of their greatest growth. They realized that during the night when they were alone or had no great group around them to give them advice, they were in fact able to make important decisions and do the right thing for patients. This is a boost to their confidence and a great maturation process for each physician as he goes through it.

Eben Alexander, Jr, M.D.

I was fortunate to serve my internship in a large city hospital in 1945 to 1946, and I have only fond memories of the nine months. We worked every other night and weekends, and slept but little while on duty, some nights not at all, and for $15 a month, room and board.

In my nine months I recall the following: 132 infant deliveries in three weeks, 18 in one night alone; caring for several patients with diabetic comas most of the night, doing hourly blood sugar level tests myself and giving insulin accordingly; 20 to 30 spinal taps every day for a month during a polio epidemic; grappling with a huge psychotic woman who had slipped her restraints and overturned her bed; half a dozen drug addicts with severe tetanus; an elderly man with pneumonia and meningitis and opisthotonos. I saw things I had only read about and have never seen again.

I would not trade those nine months for any like period in my life and consider my overworked internship a fantastic learning experience and the absolute highlight of my entire medical career.

William E. Nessell, M.D.

Sixteen years after my own internship, when I am called in an emergency to see a patient at three in the morning, I growl at the operator, I curse the patient, I curse his disease, I curse the night, I curse medicine, I curse the cold, and I curse my profession. There cannot be found in me the smallest drop of compassion. I desire nothing more than to live like other people . . . to just go and drive a truck.

But when I finally get there, when the patient is before me, I experience a great calm. Now there is nothing before me but the preservation of his good. And when I have done for him the best that I am capable of doing, it is then that I realize that in this world there are few rewards that can match the privilege of preserving the good of those who are sick. Then I am glad that I am not like other men. Without the experience of internship, as it is and must be, I am not sure I would get out of bed.

Anonymous

The physician is bound by laws that do not bind others. He is bound by a higher law. He is bound to function for the good of his patient. That good takes precedent over his feelings, his moods, his fatigue, his convenience, and even his compassion. If a physician is primarily concerned with the preservation of his "supportive attitude," his "compassion," he will subject the good of the patient to those needs. If he is willing to do that, he can substitute any good for the good of the patient. When his financial needs become important for the preservation of his compassion, he will substitute that also for the good of the patient.

George E. Mohun, M.D.

The practice of medicine, while it has its own philosophic bent, has very few similarities to the practice of law or a life spent in the clergy. We are hard-working pragmatists in a rapidly moving and some-times cruel world. The best preparation I know of for this is to place a capable medical school graduate in a tough internship and a tough residency. For us to believe otherwise, or to encourage our medical students and house staff to believe otherwise, denies the reality of the world in which we practice.

John H. Schwartz, M.D.

Norman Cousins raises a number of critical issues regarding the overworking of interns and the patterns of attitude and behavior that this practice reinforces. Having survived the experience of internship a number of years ago, and having no wish to subject my younger colleagues to the same ordeal, I applaud Mr. Cousins' attempt to get the medical profession to examine critically some of its sacred cows.

I would have to say that in years of asking the same questions of hospital administrators and clinical department chairmen I have never received a clear or adequate explanation of exactly what the young physician, his patients, or even the medical profession gain from the experience of practicing medicine while subjected to numbing fatigue. Obviously the lack of a clear explanation has hardly acted as a deterrent.

Nils M. P. Daulaire, M.D.

If Mr Cousins abolished the internship, what would be put in its place? The experiment of abolishing the internship was tried in psychiatry from 1970 to 1977. It produced compassionate psychiatrists who had not learned to function as physicians. It was found necessary to reinstitute a mini-internship, a four-month period in the first year of training in which psychiatrists could attempt to learn to be physicians before they learned to become specialists. Although this period is insufficient in duration and in the degree of clinical responsibility offered to produce the necessary result, the restoration demonstrates the failure of the attempt to do without it.

Anonymous

"Seeing patients under conditions of pressure and fatigue" is not limited to time spent during the internship. This occurs as well in the practice of most physicians caring for patients. "Feelings of resentment ... toward a patient who has a propensity for feeling his sharpest pains at 3 a.m." and hopes that a patient will die before one arrives are also not limited to interns. While he is still under the supervision of senior physicians, an intern is taught not to act on these feelings and hopes but to act in a compassionate manner regardless of his personal feelings or comfort.

It is not clear to me whether Mr. Cousins believes that physicians should never experience these feelings and stresses or whether they should never learn to cope with them—to "desensitize" themselves to them.

Lewis S. Glickman, M.D.

Although the internship may dull some unspecified "sensitivities," it helps develop other important clinical sensitivities. The only way to learn to care for patients (using "care" in the broadest definition) is to care for them—under supervision, but with enough freedom to make decisions and to be responsible for their consequences. During the day there are other physicians to consult or to rely on. At night there is a much greater "range of motion." The internship is crucial to the development of clinical judgment—the trusting of hunches, the occasional mistrusting of laboratory data, and the inclination to pursue another direction in diagnosis or therapy, which makes a physician into a superior clinician.

Furthermore, it is reasonable to expect that this clinical judgment be formed, and practiced, when the physician is tired. A physician must be able to respond semiautomatically in emergency situations, such as cardiac arrest, massive gastrointestinal hemorrhage, pulmonary edema, or severe arterial lacerations. He must know exactly what to do without needing to think about it. The fact is that major errors are rarely made because of physician fatigue; they are usually made from ignorance or poor clinical judgment and would not have been prevented by daylight or by sleep. I do not personally know of any major errors made, or of any malpractice suits for action taken, by tired interns.

Cousins asks, "How does the internship prepare the physician for the 'realities'?" Perhaps the first reality is that a physician must place the needs and interest of the patient above his or her own. This is what physicians "profess" to do and what we must continue to do if we are to remain a profession. The internship, more than any other phase of medical education, teaches this responsibility. Medicine is not a 9-to-5 job!

Daniel J. Fink, M.D.

The conditioning of the internship year has apparently great value. Medicine is not a 9-to-5 job; it is a job requiring, on an average, 55 to 80 hours per week for most practicing physicians. After an internship this seems like a holiday to most of them the rest of their lives.

Laurie E. Rennie, M.D.

Finally, it should be commented that if Mr. Cousins wishes to pontificate on American medicine, he should acquire a better data base than random discussions that are followed by sweeping generalizations. He should test his conclusions against the realities with which we in medicine struggle. In particular, his implication that the rigors of internship produce physicians who are not supportive and compassionate is nothing more than an uneducated opinion. Is an intensive year of training too much to ask of one who will be entrusted with his fellow citizen's lives?

William Meggs, M.D. Ph.D.

I could not agree more with Mr. Cousins' description of the internship year. The internship was the most hideous year of my life, and there was no need for it to have been that way. I hope that Mr. Cousins' article will stimulate others in the medical profession to "come out of the closet" and express their justifiable resentment that this anachronism still persists. The analogy to a year-long fraternity hazing is most apt!

Richard J. Steckel, M.D.

I express my sincere gratitude for bringing these facts to your readers' attention. I have gone through it for seven years of my life and I know what it is.

I am sure whoever solves this problem will be the great name in medical history.

Arundev D. Desai, M.D.

NORMAN COUSINS RESPONDS

I have been asked to comment on the mail generated by the article on the limitations and hazards of medical internship (1981; 245:377). At a rough guess, I would say that the mail ran 60 to 40 against the general thrust of the article. Pro or con, the letters seemed to me to fall into the following categories:

1. *Rites of Passage.*   The argument here is that aspiring physicians should be prepared to undergo a reasonable degree of hardship in their ascent to a profession built on a tradition of personal sacrifice. Since medicine is dedicated to healing and the alleviation of human suffering, the training of physicians should emphasize the subordination of their personal comforts and perquisites. This is a powerful argument, one that I am bound to respect, especially when advanced by physicians whose own careers are completely consistent with that viewpoint. I do not see, however, that this tradition would be seriously weakened if it took into account the health needs of the interns and not just the patients.

2. *Conditioning.*   This argument, closely related to the first, holds that internship is a useful introduction to the kind of life that the physician is about to enter. It is said that long hours, unremitting

tensions, badgering by patients, and inadequate rest and relaxation go with the franchise.

It seems to me that perhaps this argument had greater validity a quarter century or more ago, when house calls in the middle of the night were more prevalent than they are today. The decline of the little black bag is the result not so much of the reluctance of the physician to leave his office as it is of the increasingly sovereign role of modern medical technology. The modern symbol of medical treatment today is no longer the stethoscope, the tongue depressor, or the blood pressure gauge but computerized equipment and laboratory procedures.

3. *The Curriculum Factor.*   An impressive number of letters opposing current internship policies contend that the actual hospital experiences of interns are much too haphazard. A strong argument is made that internship training should be carefully planned and programmed so that the new physicians will be assured of systematic exposure to the widest possible range of cases. It is not necessarily true, these correspondents point out, that a hospital provides an assured supply of medical problems and challenges to all interns equally. Current internship policy would be strengthened, it is argued, if the schedules of new physicians were specifically and carefully arranged to assure the widest possible training. This calls for an increased administrative burden but it is thought that the need is sufficiently important to warrant the extra effort.

4. *The Hidden Agenda.*   An impressive number of correspondents contend that the entire debate is somewhat academic in view of the fact that the justification for current internship policies is less philosophic than economic. All the arguments about tradition and hardship are largely irrelevant, it is said, in light of the dependence of hospitals on low-cost labor performed by interns. Thus, long hours are seen not as essential training so much as a way of providing the hospital with a continuing and assured supply of specialized services at low cost.

It seems reasonable to me to suggest that a comprehensive study of this particular aspect of the general problem be undertaken within the profession. The recent American Medical Association study of medical school curricula is a useful model, in terms of its organization and authority.

5. *Who Shall Sleep?*   Few aspects of the controversy are more fascinating than those relating to the sleepy intern. There was much

argument but little consensus on how long an intern could go without sleep and still perform creditably. Some of the letter writers contended they could get along very well with three or four hours of sleep, and they therefore saw no reason why all interns shouldn't be able to do the same. Supposedly, the Chinese don't bet on horse races because it has long been known that one horse can run faster than another. Obviously, some physicians are better able than others to think clearly and effectively under circumstances of serious sleep deprivation. It is pointless and anecdotal, therefore, for some physicians to defend the 32-hour shift on the basis of their personal experiences. In matters of human illness, we deal with enough uncertainty without adding hazards imposed by mandated sleep deprivation of physicians, variable though the capacity of the individual may be. The law imposes standard tests against drunken driving, even though some people can hold their liquor better than others. So long as innocent third parties can be affected, the law is unwilling to take chances.

There may be no simple procedures comparable to the breath-balloon for drunken drivers, to determine whether it is risky to allow some and not other sleep-deprived physicians to attend to critical cases. Enough is known, however, about the consequences of sleep deprivation to draw up policies based on minimum rather than maximum tolerances. The finest resource of the physician is his ability to make accurate judgments at critical times. Anything that impairs the making of such judgments should be as unacceptable as the lowering of standards in national tests for the purpose of accommodating individual cases.

Here, too, it may be useful to appoint a study commission for the purpose of drawing up essential criteria. For in the final analysis, internship policies must be based not on the needs of the intern or the hospital but on the requirements of effective and safe patient care.

6. *Vital Exceptions.* It was called to my attention that a number of teaching hospitals have already initiated important reforms in the training of interns. It was embarrassing to me to learn that I had been unaware of changes instituted here at UCLA. In the Family Practice department at UCLA, the governing principle behind these changes is that interns should not be coddled but neither should they be required to treat patients under conditions of fatigue or undue stress. So far as can be ascertained, this modification of the program works out well for all concerned.

I am grateful to all those who expressed their views, either to the editor of *JAMA* or to me directly. Their comments have given me an increased awareness of the complexities of this matter, just as they have given me an increased respect for the large number of physicians who think more in terms of moral commitment than of personal advantage.

Stress During the Internship Year

Joel E. Dimsdale

INTRODUCTION

Generations of physicians have regarded the internship as a singularly stressful period in their medical training; nevertheless, the stresses of internship have been relatively ignored as compared with the intense focus on stresses encountered by the medical student. This silence regarding the tasks of internship, its stresses, and indeed its rational planning is an interesting phenomenon. In conducting a survey of standard medical history texts, I was unable to find a single reference to "interns" in the indices.[1-5] In the existing literature about internship, stress is rarely addressed directly, although some writers have alleged that the internship is a time of severe exploitation filled with psychological stress, anxiety, depression, fears of incompetence, and exhaustion.[6-13] This relative paucity of information about intern stress is striking because the internship is a time of major change.

The term "intern" itself is an interesting choice for this training period. According to the Oxford English Dictionary, an intern is an "inmate," one who is confined "within the limits of a country, district, or place."[14] How different this is from the term "student" (derived from *studeo*, meaning to be eager), or "resident" (one who rests). If etymology has anything to offer in elucidating the fate of the intern, it would appear that the intern is a rather ambivalently esteemed person.

I wish to thank the friends and colleagues who participated in this study for their candor and eloquence. I also acknowledge with appreciation Thomas P. Hackett and Kenneth Kauvar for their comments and criticism.

I have interviewed a cohort of interns and organized their comments according to the above themes. Because the group was so expressive, I will quote them extensively. Because of the small sample it is important to emphasize that these are tentative observations meant only to stimulate discussion and inquiry into this important but strangely neglected field. In the absence of a substantial literature on this topic, it seemed more appropriate to delineate the broad outlines of the problem as opposed to the details of the prevalence of various stresses.

METHODS

A semi-structured interview was designed and pretested on three first-year medical residents. Interns personally known to the author were informed about the purpose of the study and were asked to participate. Twelve of 22 medical interns at a university teaching hospital were approached for study; all agreed to participate. Most of the sample was male (11 out of 12) and married (8 out of 12). Being chosen to participate in this study was not contingent on either outspoken criticism or enthusiastic support of the internship or the hospital but merely a working acquaintance with the author. All subjects were interviewed once during their internship for approximately 1½ hours. The interviews were taperecorded and later transcribed.

RESULTS

I have divided the material into three overlapping categories: general physical health, social and lifestyle changes, and subjective emotional distress.

Physical Health

Three-quarters of the interns developed a weight change of at least 2 kilograms (one intern lost 5 kilograms in the first two weeks of internship!). One-third of them experienced increased minor gastrointestinal difficulties such as diarrhea, nausea, constipation; a few complained of an increase in headaches. The events triggering a

TABLE 1   Health complaints during internship

Complaint	Number of interns ($N = 12$)*
Major illness	0
Weight change	9
Gastrointestinal symptoms	
Worse	5
No change	3
Better	0
Headaches	
Worse	2
No change	6
Better	1
Sleep deprivation	7
Hospital dreams	10
Sexual functioning	
Worse	9
No change	1
Better	2
Ignorance of blood pressure	7
Use of opiates, amphetamines, barbiturates	0
Alcohol	
Increased	1
No change	5
Decreased	6
Marijuana	
Increased	0
No change	5
Decreased	6

*Some interns did not answer all questions; $N \neq 12$ for all categories.

headache or GI upset were generally periods of increased tension, such as the first day on a new rotation or conflicts with a resident or attending physician. Illness causing absence from work for at least two days was very rare. The incidence of minor illnesses such as colds seemed unchanged, although some interns complained that the duration of minor illnesses was longer during their internship year (see Table 1).

Most subjects complained of sleep deprivation. The great majority became accustomed to chronic sleep deprivation by learning simply not to expect much physical exuberance and learning the art of taking quick cat-naps. Sleep, when it did come, was disturbed by hospital-related dreams in over three-quarters of the sample. These dreams generally involved treating moribund patients.

> I really wouldn't be aware of it at the time but I would be dreaming about somebody arresting somewhere, get out of bed, and my wife would ask what the hell I was doing.

> I dream a lot about the hospital, dream of resuscitating people. I know the other day my wife woke me up for dinner, tapped me on the shoulder and I turned and said to her, "Is he in failure?"

Sexual functioning was diminished in three-fourths of the group. The married interns seemed to experience this more than the single interns.

One of my health assessment questions concerned recent blood pressure. To my surprise, I found that over half of the group had no idea what their blood pressure was. Despite an ideology favoring early detection and treatment of illness, their attitude regarding themselves seemed to be one of denial of vulnerability to illness, a problem encountered in other physician groups.[15]

There was no self-report of any continuing pattern of drug abuse. In college and medical school most had experimented with marijuana and a few smoked it rather regularly; however, during the internship they rarely used marijuana. Alcohol intake was decreased in 6, increased in 1, and unchanged in 5 interns.

Social and Lifestyle Changes

Half of the group made major geographical moves to begin their internship. Particularly among the movers there was considerable mourning for old locations, medical school, friends, and hobbies. Some interns deferred unpacking books and belongings for months after the start of internship, claiming initially that time pressures were too intense but later stating that they didn't feel "at home" yet and wanted to be ready to move again. After about six months of internship, this "mourning" turned into "nostalgia." To the movers, the city remained alien throughout most of the internship (see Table 2).

Many complained of limited friendships and social ties. Their social interaction seemed limited to their internship group or other hospital personnel. They missed having friends outside of the hospital and time to pursue well-developed hobbies.

TABLE 2   Social and lifestyle changes

Change	Number of interns ($N = 12$)
Geographical move	5
Restricted friendship and hobbies	9
Decreased physical activity	7
Intimate relationship	
Severely jeopardized	3
Moderate conflict	3
No change	4
Better relationship	1
Uninvolved	1

Many interns were concerned about the lack of time for physical exercise. Most of them had been active athletically throughout medical school. They found that such physical activity was relaxing, enabling them to meet with friends and keeping them in reasonably good shape.

> It really bothers me. I used to be in good shape. All day I see these wrecks of patients who are in poor shape and I realize I'm moving in that direction too; the old arteries are just silting up.

One-fourth of the interns who were married or who had a close intimate relationship were considering a separation or had completed a separation. One-fourth complained that the internship put moderate stresses on the relationship because of their spouse's dissatisfaction with the time demands, their limited vitality during their days off, and their absorption with hospital-related topics when they came home. Those interns having children found that they had little time to spend with them.

> My five-year-old boy knew what he did *not* want to become after I had been an intern for a month.

Emotional Distresses

The first days of the internship were uniquely trying. Those interns who had worked in this hospital as medical students were at an advantage to their newly arrived peers. The newly arrived interns complained that the orientation—which consisted of filling out numerous forms, welcome speeches, distributing vacation schedules, and a brief discussion of the mechanics of the hospital—was inadequate. Numerous pragmatic points such as hospital floor plans, mechanics of patient transport, and ways of filling out laboratory forms were discussed in short order (see Table 3).

In the first days almost everyone felt extremely incompetent medically and had the secret conviction that "either the Selection Committee or the internship match computer made a mistake; I really shouldn't be here." The first days also brought the personal experience of medical responsibility, embarrassment, and patient death.

> My first patient was a horror because when I got back the set of electrolytes, I couldn't even remember what the significance was. Not only that, the patient had turned out to have acute renal failure and I thought he had gastroenteritis.
>
> I had a line of unattractive patients, aesthetically and disease-wise; they were a pain in the ass. Seeing them day after day—this one pulled out her IV—I got anxious, depressed, annoyed—"what am I doing, I would ask myself." One was a 28-year-old woman who would voluntarily vomit on demand. She was passive aggressive, no veins left. Another was an alcoholic who was depressed. Another was a lady with valvular disease who was depressed and all she did at night was scream and I couldn't give her pain meds; next was a fat diabetic lady with septicemia and whose IV kept infiltrating—none of whom seemed worth saving and all of whom were burdening me beyond my belief with their individual problems.

TABLE 3   Emotional distress

Complaint	Number of interns ($N = 12$)
Initial feelings of incompetence	11
Dissatisfaction with pay or on-call schedule	1
Major interpersonal conflict	8
Depressive symptoms	8
Suicidal ideation	1
Unawareness of hospital suicides	8
Most stressful life experience	
Internship	0
Early academic achievement	10
Other	2
Blossoming experience	10

Although the sense of profound incompetency soon disappeared, most of the group did not feel competent for four to six months.

In this hospital, as in most others, the interns' vacation schedule was set rigidly without any input from the affected intern. Those interns who were assigned an early vacation found their newly won and rather tenuous sense of competency dashed. They returned from their vacation fearing that they had forgotten all they had learned in internship or in medical school and dreading the prospect of ten more months of internship without a vacation.

Learning to handle the flood of information efficiently was especially trying.

> I can remember I had a patient in EW. I went down to see him, was doing the write up and got another case. I was in the middle of writing the history—the other case was even more complicated, had to be seen immediately. So I dropped the first work up I was doing, ran downstairs for the next one. It turned out I got two more after I had begun the first one and hadn't written down either of them. It was about 11:00 p.m. At that time I began to sort of lose track of who had the S4 and who had the S3 and the physicals began to run together in my mind and I began to just sort of overload—the feeling that I wasn't actually able to write down what I had actually seen or had done during that day—and I realized I had to become much quicker and set up a sort of system with priorities during the day—do the things that were most urgent first and to be kind of quick on your feet."

There was little criticism of pay or on-call schedule; the group appeared to accept these as "givens." What really troubled them was interpersonal discord. The interns came from medical school eager to work with perfectly rational colleagues and patients. They were unprepared to deal with fallible human beings and either responded with rage at the shortcomings of other personnel or, like brave Achilles, sulked in their tents when they were the target of another's unpleasant idiosyncrasies. It is hard work navigating in the hospital world, work that requires tact, humility, and tolerance. Months of painful experience preceded the emergence of these necessary skills.

> The nursing staff had been told that the guy was a DO NOT RESUSCITATE and then when he looked sick, the nursing staff completely ignored him. Finally I was asked to look at him when he was kind of in an agonal state, and then I started treating his

heart. On rounds the next day, I got the "why didn't you realize the guy probably had a dig toxic arrhythmia?" I went home, thinking it was a disaster, that this guy had died too early because of me, that I had done a terrible thing. The next day I had a confrontation with the nurse on duty. She had told my resident that she had told me the instant the patient looked bad and that was a lie, and I blew up at her. I was so anxious, I made a federal case out of it, pulling temperature sheets. About an hour later the assistant resident called me aside and talked with me on the lawn and said "look, you're not getting things together here. It doesn't matter whether you were wrong or right. You have to realize that if you blow up at people they are going to get scared of you; and if something really terrible happens, they are going to be scared to call you."

Interns became extremely distressed when a superior made a particularly harsh, denigrating remark. If the insult was accompanied by "public shaming," the distress was naturally intensified. While this was not a common experience, it had a dramatic impact on the intern's still tenuous self-confidence.

I had Dr. V. for attending for a month. He is huge like a bear and was always springing questions on me in front of other people, not teaching me, you know, but testing me. The whole period I was sick as a dog with nausea and vomiting.

I get really depressed when somebody makes me feel like "little boy inferior." I had missed a liver mass and everybody laughed at me. The resident in his infinite wisdom declared my actions were folly. You know, there are nice ways to tell people things and there are not so nice ways.

Friction also occurred between interns and nurses or other hospital employees. The interns tended to regard themselves as the hardworking "heart" of the hospital. They were exhausted by their schedule and yet derived some pleasure from knowing how hard they worked. This led them frequently to make envious comparisons with laboratory personnel, X-ray, etc. Particularly at the beginning of the internship, the nurses were regarded with ambivalence. Interns wanted help from them but were embarrassed to ask; nurses wanted help from the interns but resented their transience.

Half the internship group complained of depressive symptoms such as feeling moody, blue, loss of appetite, hopelessness and, occasionally, suicidal ideation. Many complained of feeling "imprisoned," particularly in the winter time.

> I would wake up early and go into the hospital while it was dark.
> There I would work for thirty-six hours surrounded by the same
> patients and other exhausted friends. At the end of that I would
> go home and it was still dark. I started to feel as if I were in a labor
> camp, like Solzhenitzyn talks about, boxed in.

Depression was a taboo subject among the interns. While
interns were quite ready to vent off anger and frustration with their
friends, and at least sometimes ready to talk about anxiety and
discouragement, they kept their depression to themselves.

> I feel I'm different than when I walked into that EW the first day.
> I'm not sure I like the way I'm different. It's not been a good year
> for me [voice cracks]. It's true that I'm more confident about
> things, but it's been so stressful. I feel tired all the time. I feel torn,
> don't feel myself. I used to know what I wanted, used to feel that
> everything is right. I don't feel that way now. All I feel is, uhmm,
> kind of sick.

They were only faintly aware of depression in others. One of the
questions on the interview asked whether the intern knew of any
house staff at the hospital who had been upset enough to
contemplate suicide. It was a timely question; the year prior to this
study saw an unusual tragedy—two completed suicides and one
attempted suicide by house staff from other departments of the
hospital. Despite a rich gossip mill and much interaction with interns
and residents from other services, these suicides were "unknown" to
two-thirds of the interns. When confronted with the news that
suicides had occurred, some interns became defensively belligerent.

> What do you mean, suicide? You have to be wrong. If there was a
> suicide, I would know about it. Look, we have these rosters with
> everybody's picture on it. They're all here, I swear; they're still all
> there.

Hospitals have intricate webs of rumor and gossip; newcomers learn
rapidly by having the example of predecessors held up for emulation
or warning. They learn about idiosyncracies of attending staff and
about the various states of disarray in colleagues' lives. It is
intriguing that so painful a topic as the suicides of two young
physicians was either not "transmitted" or not "received" by the
interns. The interns deal with their depression and that of their
friends by developing a large blind spot regarding the whole topic.

While the data indicate that the internship is an extremely
stressful period, all the interns stated that they had experienced far

worse stress earlier in their lives. In some cases these "worst experiences" resulted from the loss of beloved family members; however, most of the group localized these stresses to past crises of academic achievement in medical school, college, or even high school. One loses sight of the length and meaning of the intern's career as an academic competitor. Twenty years of training and achievement are necessary before the intern can arrive and experience his internship. For most of the group, the early academic competition and achievement pressure were far more taxing than the internship, perhaps because the individual was younger, more vulnerable, and less mature at such points.

> My hardest time came in applying for college. I got turned down by Princeton, my "safe school." I had not heard at that point from the others, but I felt like, that was it, at 17 years of age I was a washout, an academic mediocrity.

DISCUSSION

Each intern I interviewed experienced his internship in unique terms, but there are certain common themes. This group appeared to accept as "given" the rigorous call schedule and low salary. Some even thought that every other night on call was superior to every third night on call. Most felt that such strenuous training was necessary for the practice of medicine; as one intern put it, "there is no picnic without ants." The interns' physical health was relatively unaffected. Sleep and sexual functioning were noticeably curtailed. Most of the marriages were stressed during the internship, but only a few were in severe turmoil. The loss of time to pursue hobbies and friends outside the hospital was resented. Depression, sometimes of rather alarming proportion, was uniformly ignored.

The most stressful situation involved disagreements with coworkers, nurses, residents, and attendings. Interns were surprisingly unprepared to deal with irrational behavior, either in patients or hospital staff. Despite all the unpleasantness involved in internship, not one subject thought the internship was the most stressful event in his life. Many found the internship a time of blossoming despite its hardships. The thrill of finally "arriving" to practice medicine, of beginning financial self-sufficiency, or observing one's rapid acquisition of clinical knowledge, all combined to make the internship a time of excitement and growth as well as stress.

It would be presumptuous of me to make specific recommendations for the modification of internship on the basis of this small sample from one hospital. However, at the risk of going out on a limb, I would like to offer some tentative opinions. Some of these stresses seem unavoidable because of the very nature of internship. Some, however, could be ameliorated by more rational planning of the internship itself. Although the intern's pay, call schedule, and life outside of the hospital have been liberalized in the past 30 years, certain commonly found administrative aspects of the internship, such as arbitrary vacation schedules and abbreviated orientation, persist and appear needlessly disruptive. Some of these administrative details appear easily modifiable; some would require planning so extensive that it is perhaps naive to expect changes. Some stress may also be attributed to a pattern of medical school education that does not emphasize adequately preparation for the human tasks of internship. It is not that the medical student does not learn his anatomy or his medicine; it is that he is not taught to perceive the difficulties or to practice the skills necessary for functioning in a complex bureaucracy.

REFERENCES

1. C. Singer, E. Underwood, *A Short History of Medicine*. Oxford University Press, New York, 1962.

2. F. Garrison, *Introduction to the History of Medicine*, 3rd Ed. Saunders Company, Philadelphia, 1924.

3. A. Castiglioni, *A History of Medicine*. Knopf & Co., New York, 1941.

4. F. Packard, *History of Medicine in the United States*. Hafner Publishing Co., New York, 1963.

5. L. Morton, *Garrison and Morton's Medical Bibliography*, 2nd Ed. Argosy Bookstore, New York, 1954.

6. E. Bassuk, C. Nadelson, "A Dilemma in Medical Education," *J. Med. Educ.* 47: 894–900, 1972.

7. J. Duffy, "Suicides by Physicians in Training," *J. Med. Educ.* 43: 1196, 1968.

8. C. Coste, "Stress: The Dark Side of Training," *New Physician*, November 1976, pp. 38–39.

9. J. Duffy, "The Emotional Health of Physicians," *Annals of Internal Medicine* 69: 1319–22, 1968.

10. R. Heller, L. Robertson, J. Alpert, "Health Care of House Officers," *NEJM* 277: 907–910, 1967.

11. R. Friedman, D. Kornfeld, T. Bigger, "Psychological Problems Associated with Sleep Deprivation in Interns," *J. Med. Educ.* 48: 436–441, 1973.

12. N. McAlister, "House Staffs on Strike," Letter to the Editor, *NEJM* 294: 1349, 1976.

13. R. Friedman, T. Bigger, D. Kornfeld, "The Intern and Sleep Loss," *NEJM* 285: 201–203, 1971.

14. *Oxford English Dictionary*. Oxford University Press, Oxford, 1961, p. 409.

15. J. Sharpe, W. Smith, "Physician, Heal Thyself: Comparison on Findings in Periodic Health Examinations of Physicians and Executives," *JAMA* 182: 234–237, 1962.

House Officer Stress Syndrome

Gary W. Small

The well-known risks of internship and residency—depression, marital problems, alcohol abuse, and the like—actually may represent features of a house officer stress syndrome. Merklin and Little have described a "beginning psychiatry training syndrome" characterized by anxiety, depression, and psychosomatic disturbances. Seven features characterize the house officer stress syndrome: (1) episodic cognitive impairment, (2) chronic anger, (3) pervasive cynicism, (4) family discord, (5) depression, (6) suicidal ideation and suicide, and (7) substance abuse. Although usually benign, the first four features of the syndrome—cognitive impairment, anger, cynicism, and family discord—occur in nearly all house officers. Those severely affected may also suffer from the more malignant features—depression, suicidal ideation, and substance abuse.

CHARACTERISTIC FEATURES

1. Episodic Cognitive Impairment

Cognition, the mental process of comprehension, judgment, memory, and reasoning, is a prerequisite to adequate performance by a house officer. Episodic impairment in cognition, however, occurs among house officers. Friedman and associates[3,4] tested cognition in 14 interns who had each remained awake for approximately 30 hours. In comparison with their performance when rested, the interns deprived of sleep showed significant impairment in their ability to recognize arrhythmias on electrocardiograms. Transient mood changes accompanied their intellectual deterioration, including increased sadness, irritability, anger, and inappropriate affect usually associated with black humor. While some interns feared that the damage incurred from sleep loss would become permanent, others feared more their loss of control during long periods without sleep.

2. Chronic Anger

The house officer faces extreme demands of time and energy. He or she experiences a natural response to these demands—resentment. Early in training a chronic low-grade elevation of anger analogous to a low-grade fever may develop. Actual outbursts of rage erupt infrequently and probably correlate with the amount of sleep deprivation.[3,4] House officer slang suggests these daily feelings of anger. Housestaff often talk not of patients but of "gomers" (the acronym for "get out of my emergency room"), "turkeys," and "crocks."[5] The middle-of-the-night patient, the "hit in the pit," might get "dumped" onto someone else's service but often "bounces" back to the original intern or resident. In the context of training and out of the patient's earshot, this slang provides a way for the house officer to discharge at least some anger. The house officer directs anger not only toward patients but also toward supervisors, colleagues, family, friends and, finally, toward the self.

3. Pervasive Cynicism

House officer slang exemplifies an intensification of cynicism. The cynic, believing that selfish interests motivate people, shows detachment and toughness when relating to others. During the course of training, the house officer's motivation tends to shift from wanting to help others in distress to wanting to protect his or her own limited time and energy. For example, at the end of a consultation note about a chronically ill patient, a resident may add, "P.S. My clinic is full." Studies of medical students indicate that cynicism increasingly intermingles with idealism and humanitarianism during medical school.[6] This cynicism appears to be a situational response to the stresses of medical education rather than a manifestation of an established personality trait. Cynicism persists throughout postgraduate training and perhaps allows the house officer to cope with the barrage of frustrations faced each day.

4. Family Discord

Vaillant and associates[7] reported that nearly half of the 47 physicians in their study experienced marital maladjustment, i.e., a sense of instability in the relationship, sexual dissatisfaction, or consideration of divorce. This finding held true in particular for physicians with primary responsibility for patient care. The house officer spending a considerable amount of time providing direct patient care, therefore, may be especially susceptible to marital maladjustment. Whether or not a house officer's marriage ends in divorce, extreme demands on time and energy inevitably interfere with family life. After working 80 or more hours a week, there may be little energy left for the demands of interpersonal relationships.

5. Depression

Clinically significant depression, the most common psychiatric disorder, affects an estimated 15% of the general population at some time in life.[8] Women suffer from depression more frequently than men by a 2:1 ratio. Among practicing physicians, women may also be more susceptible. Welner and associates[9] found that 51% of the 111 women physicians in their study suffered from depression, a significantly higher rate than that found in a control group of women holding Ph.D.s who were matched for age, marital status, and race.

Valko and Clayton[10] studied depression in house officers. They found that 30% (16) of 53 medical and surgical house officers became depressed during internship. Depression was diagnosed, by the Feighner criteria, as a month or more of a dysphoric mood with at least four of the following symptoms: fatigue, appetite disorder, loss of interest, sleep disturbance, impaired concentration, feelings of guilt or self-reproach, thoughts of death or suicide, and agitation or retardation. These depressive episodes averaged five months in duration and generally occurred at the beginning of internship on those services with the longest working hours. Marital discord, a frequent accompaniment of depression, often was seen as a clue to the onset of a depressive episode.

6. Suicidal Ideation and Suicide

Each year, a number of physicians equal to that of an average-sized medical school graduating class commit suicide.[11] Male physicians commit suicide at a rate 1.15 times that of the overall male population, whereas the rate for female physicians is three times that expected for the general female population.[12] The suicide rate for house officers has never been reported and is difficult to estimate. In the Valko and Clayton study,[10] the thought of suicide, more common than the act, was experienced by four of the 16 depressed interns—i.e., 8% of the 53 interns. Since suicidal ideation usually indicates depression, recognition and treatment of depression in house officers could prevent some suicides.

7. Substance Abuse

The California State Board of Medical Examiners has estimated that at some point in their careers 1% to 2% of California physicians abuse narcotics.[13] In a 25-year period, the New York Bureau of Narcotic Control recorded ½% of licensed physicians in that state as addicts.[13] This rate of addiction exceeds by a factor of five the rate for American men 20 to 50 years of age. A 20-year prospective study by Vaillant and associates[13] showed that a group of 45 physicians took more tranquilizers, sedatives, and stimulants than 90 matched controls.

Availability of drugs and the common practice of self-administration of medications perhaps contribute to drug abuse by physicians. Heller and associates[14] reported that self-administration of medications is indeed commonplace among physicians: 39% of the house officers in their study assumed full responsibility for antibiotic treatment for themselves. It seems unlikely that house officers use addictive drugs at a rate comparable to their personal use of antibiotics. Regardless of its actual prevalence, drug abuse by house officers has repercussions. Morbidity and mortality often accompany substance abuse: 20% of physicians' suicides are associated with drug abuse, 40% with alcohol abuse.[11] According to the American Medical Association's obituaries, by my count seven house officers died in 1978 from drug overdoses.

ETIOLOGY

What causes the house officer stress syndrome? The precise relationship between stressful aspects of training and the features of the syndrome is unclear. All house officers face stresses. These stresses, moreover, may ensure clinical competence as much as they contribute to features of the syndrome. Among others, the following stresses contribute to the syndrome.

Sleep Deprivation

Work schedules requiring interns and residents to be on call range from every other night to every sixth night; most programs schedule duty every third night. Sometimes trainees work even longer hours. For example, Friedman and associates[4] studied a group of interns at a major teaching hospital in New York City where, during the early 1970s, house officers often stayed awake for a call period of 60 hours during one weekend. Their study showed that prolonged sleep deprivation causes impairment of cognition and affect. Sleep deprivation, therefore, probably contributes to cognitive impairment, chronic anger, and may prove to contribute to other symptoms as well.

Excessive Work Load

Rhoads[15] reported 14 case histories of professionals suffering from overwork. These accountants, lawyers, and physicians attempted to cope with fatigue and an inability to concentrate by forcing themselves to continue performing their appointed tasks. Most of them recovered following an enforced vacation period. Although few of the 14 suffered from sleep deprivation, many of their symptoms closely resembled several features of the syndrome. A house officer's extreme amount of work may therefore contribute to the syndrome regardless of the degree of sleep deprivation. The excessive work load of training may not only contribute to stress but may also ensure maximum learning, assuming of responsibility, and habit formation.

Patient Care Responsibility

From the first day of internship the house officer assumes direct and, at times, full responsibility for patient care. In a study of 47 physicians compared with a group of 79 matched nonphysician controls, Vaillant and associates[7] noted that "Physicians, especially those involved in direct patient care, were more likely than controls to have relatively poor marriages, to use drugs and alcohol heavily, and to obtain psychotherapy." This study suggests that direct patient care could contribute to family discord and substance abuse, although Vaillant did not delineate which aspects of direct patient care (work load, responsibility per se, or some other factor) contribute to psychological vulnerability.

Bosk[16] discussed the different kinds of errors house officers make when caring for patients. Attending physicians expect the trainee to make certain mistakes, particularly technical errors related to the learning of new skills. They forgive house officers for such errors but expect them to remember them and to make fewer errors over time. Intensive training, the rapid acquisition of skills, and "learning by doing" result in these inevitable errors. Housestaff often learn by following the aphorism "See one, do one, teach one," a method whereby habits of practice are formed. If the house officer already suffers from depression or low self-esteem, repeated errors are a source of additional stress.

Perpetually Changing Work Conditions

Since most teaching programs operate on a rotating basis, house officers find themselves on a new floor or ward every month of two; at Massachusetts General Hospital medical interns rotate to a new service every 18 to 36 days. Once house officers become comfortable in a new working situation—for example, by knowing where to find number 19 butterflies and how to get along with the charge nurse—they move on to the next service. Some programs use a team system with three or four house officers working together in a group sharing clinical responsibilities. With this system, the question is: Will the house officer get along with a new team of colleagues, a group he or she will see more often than anyone else in life during that rotation? Unreliable or interpersonally troublesome house officers generate additional work and vexation for their teammates. One major concern about constantly changing work conditions is whether house officers will team up with others unable to pull their own weight.

Peer Competition

Competition is a reality of medical training. Many teaching programs have a pyramidal structure in which only the best performers advance to the next year of training; the less talented transfer to less prestigious programs. Teaching rounds often provide an opportunity for colleagues to outdo one another. Competition motivates the house officer to do a better job; when excessive, however, it may lead to social isolation. In a work setting incorporating a team approach, cooperation is crucial for optimal patient care. Excessive competition might be detrimental to trainees as well as to patients.

PREVENTION AND MANAGEMENT

Traditionally, internship and residency have been viewed as initiation rites into professional ranks. These years of postgraduate training have been a proving ground for young physicians. The question is, What is proved? Since many stresses of training are necessary and probably productive, the real question is how to make sure these stresses remain productive rather than become destructive.

Improved Work Conditions

Several studies recommend a decrease in the duration of work shifts[4,10,17] or a reduction in the number of routine daily tasks that have minimal training value.[18] Such changes could reduce the personal and economic loss attributed to impaired performance by fatigued housestaff. The studies by Friedman and associates[3,4] on sleep-deprived interns indicate that fatigued house officers make cognitive errors and perhaps should not remain awake for 30 consecutive hours. Research on state-dependent learning, however, suggests that learning during periods of sleep deprivation may have some value during training.[19] This research has shown that if subjects learn in a drug-induced state, their retention is improved when they are in the same drug-induced state for testing. This phenomenon appears to hold true for sleeping states as well.[20] If this research applies to states of sleep deprivation, then information learned during periods of sleep deprivation may be remembered only during similar sleep-deprived periods and not during restful mental states. A house officer would thus need to learn clinical skills in both sleep-deprived and restful states in order to be prepared for emergencies in either situation. Controversy continues as to how much sleep deprivation can be tolerated and how much might be useful in attaining clinical competence.

Humor

As Nietzsche observed, "Man alone suffers so excruciatingly in the world that he was compelled to invent laughter."[21] Confronted with sickness, death, and failure, house officers naturally respond with some form of humor. Bosk[22] suggests that gallows humor, with its detachment, resignation, helplessness, and anger, is one way in which physicians manage the uncertainty of clinical practice. Many house officers feel uncomfortable with black humor rampant in medical training. Understanding the use of humor and acknowledging its natural occurrence and its effectiveness in coping with stressful feelings might lessen the impact of the syndrome.

Support Groups

The use of small groups based on a didactic or supportive model is not new to the training of medical students. Membership size and cohesiveness appear to promote the success of these groups. Experience with such groups[23-25] suggests that they do well when leaders (1) make participation optional, (2) clarify the purpose and methods of the group, (3) arrange meetings at a convenient time and place, and (4) maintain a nonjudgmental attitude toward group members and avoid passivity and aloofness. Despite favorable subjective evaluations of such groups, no one has studied their effect on work performance or work-related stress.

In the literature, there is one description of a support group for house officers.[26] This group of pediatric interns met weekly and discussed work pressures, work-related personal problems, and feelings of anxiety and victimization. The participants experienced a reduction in competitiveness and an increased ability to cope with problems at work.

For the past three years, the department of medicine of the Massachusetts General Hospital has supported "autognosis" groups for medical house officers. According to Messner,[27] who in this context introduced the term—*auto* (self), *gnosis* (knowledge)— autognosis "includes all knowledge of the self which might be relevant to the clinician's professional activities. . . . It includes awareness of perceptions, intuition, empathy, prejudices, emotions, fantasies, traits, skills, attitudes, motivation, and other internal events and processes of the clinician." For an hour each week, six to eight medical house officers meet with a staff psychiatrist and consider patient management using the autognostic approach, which provides a cognitive and emotional framework in a supportive setting. House officers look forward to these meetings and find them valuable. The question, however, remains: Do these groups, like the other support groups described, have a measurable impact on house officers? The answer to this question awaits further study.

Psychiatric Referral

House officers severely affected by depression, suicidal thought, or substance abuse require psychiatric intervention. A house officer suffering from a major depression will experience a dysphoric mood associated with other symptoms, including insomnia, changed appetite, difficulty concentrating, decreased energy, loss of interest, feelings of guilt, thoughts of suicide, and agitation or retardation. Excessive irritability, indecisiveness, disorganization, or marital discord may also provide clues to the onset of a depressive episode. If 30% of medical interns suffer from treatable depression, as suggested by Valko and Clayton,[10] then psychiatric intervention could help a considerable number of physicians in training.

CONCLUSIONS

The house officer stress syndrome, to sumarize, is a stress response syndrome affecting most house officers. Episodic cognitive impairment, chronic anger, pervasive cynicism, and family discord characterize the benign form of the syndrome. Perhaps this benign form enhances a person's ability to learn, to function under stress, and to perform competently as a clinician. Depression, suicidal ideation, and substance abuse, the malignant features of the syndrome, require psychiatric intervention.

Despite the problems posed by the stresses of postgraduate medical training, the majority of house officers graduate as competent clinicians, able to care for their patients with technical skill and sophistication. Most survive the proving ground and no other system of training has yet been proven as effective. Nevertheless, the potentially grave consequences of the stresses of training on house officers, their patients, and their families suggest a need for further study to determine what causes the house officer stress syndrome and what specific steps can be taken to prevent it.

REFERENCES

1. Cassem NH: Internship, liberty, death and other choices. *Harvard Med Alumni Bull* 53:46–48, 1979.

2. Merklin L, Little RB: Beginning psychiatry training syndrome. *Am J Psychiatry* 124:193–197, 1967.

3. Friedman RC, Bigger JT, Kornfeld DS: The intern and sleep loss. *N Engl J Med* 285:201–203, 1971.

4. Friedman RC, Kornfeld DS, Bigger TJ: Psychological problems associated with sleep deprivation in interns. *J Med Educ* 48:436–441, 1973.

5. Reynolds RE, Bice TW: Attitudes of medical interns toward patients and health professionals. *J Health Soc Behav* 12:307–311, 1971.

6. Reinhardt AM, Gray RM: A social psychological study of attitude change in physicians. *J Med Educ* 47:112–117, 1972.

7. Vaillant GE, Sobowale NC, McArthur C: Some psychologic vulnerabilities of physicians. *N Engl J Med* 287:372–375, 1972.

8. Gelenberg AJ: Affective disorders, in Lazare A (ed): *Outpatient Psychiatry*. Baltimore, Williams & Wilkins Co, 1979, pp 370–387.

9. Welner A, Marten S, Wochnick E, et al: Psychiatric disorders among professional women. *Arch Gen Psychiatry* 36:169–173, 1979.

10. Valko RJ, Clayton PJ: Depression in internship. *Dis Nerv Syst* 36:26–29, 1975.

11. Ross M: Suicide among physicians. *Psychiatry Med* 2:189–198, 1971.

12. Steppacher RC, Mausner JS: Suicide in male and female physicians. *JAMA* 228:323–328, 1974.

13. Vaillant GE, Brighton JR, McArthur C: Physicians' use of mood-altering drugs. *N Engl J Med* 282:365–370, 1970.

14. Heller RJ, Robertson LS, Alpert JJ: Health care of house officers. *N Engl J Med* 277:907–910, 1967.

15. Rhoads JM: Overwork. *JAMA* 237:2615–2618, 1977.

16. Bosk CL: Error, rank, and responsibility, in *Forgive and Remember: Managing Medical Failure*. Chicago, University of Chicago Press, 1979, pp 35–70.

17. McManus IC, Lockwood DNJ, Cruickshank, JK: The preregistration year: Chaos by consensus. *Lancet* 1:413–416, 1977.

18. Bates EM, Moore BN: Stress in hospital personnel. *Med J Aust* 2:765–767, 1975.

19. Swanson JM, Kinsbourne M: State-dependent learning and retrieval: Methodological cautions and theoretical considerations, in Kihlstrom JF, Evans FJ (eds): *Functional Disorders of Memory*. Hillsdale, NJ, Lawrence Erlbaum Assoc, 1979, pp 275–299.

20. Evans FJ, Gustafson LA, O'Connell DN, et al: Verbally induced behavioral responses during sleep. *J Nerv Ment Dis* 150:171–187, 1970.

21. Nietzsche FW: The will to power, in Mencken HL (ed): *A New Dictionary of Quotations*. New York, Alfred A Knopf, 1942, p 654.

22. Bosk CL: Occupational rituals in patient management. *N Engl J Med* 305:71–76, 1980.

23. Seguin CA: Groups in medical education. *J Med Educ* 40:281–285, 1965.

24. Cadden JJ, Flach FF, Blakeslee S, et al: Growth in medical students through group process. *Am J Psychiatry* 126:862–868, 1969.

25. Dashef SS, Espey WM. Lazarus JA: Time-limited sensitivity groups for medical students. *Am J Psychiatry* 131:287–292, 1974.

26. Siegel B, Donnelly JC: Enriching personal and professional development: The experience of a support group for interns. *J Med Educ* 53:908–914, 1978.

27. Messner E: Autognosis: Diagnosis by the use of the self, in Lazare A (ed): *Outpatient Psychiatry*. Baltimore, Williams & Wilkins Co, 1979, pp 230–237.

The Goal

Anonymous

I am the wife of a sixth-year surgical resident. My husband is in a highly selective surgical subspecialty. In a field replete with top-notch members, my husband competes and succeeds. The price of his success has been the loss of a meaningful life outside the hospital milieu. The life-and-death events that my husband handles on a daily basis with skill, dedication, and empathy perhaps have served as catalysts in his change from a loving, caring husband and father to an exhausted, passive "boarder" who only occasionally arrives home during daylight hours.

The intensity of a surgeon's training has been tradition-bound to "break the man but not his mind." Eight years ago, when we married, my husband was a medical student. I listened to him, as class president, deliver his medical school's graduation speech, and I did so with a commitment to help him become the physician he dreamed of becoming—a healer; a surgeon ("The Goal"). As president of his medical school class, as a community leader in fund-raising, and as a Big Brother volunteer, my husband remained true to himself—a person whose humanistic ideals were embodied in the way he conducted his daily life.

During the first years of his surgery training, when I was teaching emotionally disturbed children and raising our daughter, I coped, only occasionally losing sight of The Goal. Coping involved emergency room visits to local hospitals when our daughter became ill (always, it seemed, at 3 a.m. on daddy's "on-call" nights), and one Christmas Eve ER trip that I still remember vividly. The miscarriage I was having was cleaned up without more than a small dose of Demerol and some handholding from a young nurse while my obstetrician complained that it would take too long for an anesthesiologist to arrive on this holiday night (and he wanted to get home).

My husband was on call for surgery, and in his kindness as senior resident on duty, dismissed the other resident and intern, since it was a quiet night. This professional benevolence on his part and the lack of adequate staff backup left me alone that night. Although I recall having felt somewhat triumphant in knowing I could now cope with *anything* myself—even losing a child—The Goal suddenly seemed less important, as the emotional needs of our family continued to be neglected.

We endured as best we could. He, consumed in patient care and research (one of the more published residents at the medical center), while I taught school and taught his little girl to admire her daddy and understand that his growing absence was necessary to help other children who were less fortunate. And she endured. A little 4-year-old who was known by the hospital switchboard operators on a first-name basis. A 4-year old who dreamed of becoming a nurse, in hopes of seeing her daddy more. A child who loved the precious few hours every other Sunday with her daddy, hours often spent taking off his three-day-old socks and placing pillows under his head while mommy tried to feed him in bed because he was too exhausted to sit at the kitchen table.

My husband will complete his residency in June—11 years of training counting medical school. He will, I am certain, make great strides in his field. Perhaps he will remember a few of the things his family endured for his chosen professional goal. The attorney who is handling the separation informs me that starting salaries are quite high in my husband's subspecialty. I remember the loans I gladly signed during the years of training to supplement his income, to pay the rent. Child support is assured to be more than adequate, the attorney says, but because I am now in law school, my future earnings will preclude "rehabilitative" maintenance. My "rehabilitation" will involve a mending of my heart, I tell this attorney.

We made it through medical school and most of residency. We coped for a long time, in our different ways. His patients should be grateful. Their bright young surgeon has been skillfully trained but selfishly possessed by a system that forgets that behind many good residents are their families, waiting.

When the Obstetrician Gets Pregnant

Suzanne Trupin

At age 27 I was a chief resident in obstetrics and gynecology and about to have a baby. When I told one of my colleagues that I was pregnant, he put his arm around me and asked, "Do you know what is worse than having a doctor's wife as a patient?" When I shook my head, he smiled and said, "Having a doctor." He was right.

Physicians in general are troublesome, even high risk patients. They tend to think they don't need early consultations because they know it all. They dislike being tested because they know tests are uncomfortable and the results can be misleading. And they tend to take care of everyone and everything before themselves.

For the same reasons obstetricians can make some of the worst expectant mothers—and resident obstetricians the worst of the worst. To begin with, medical knowledge can heighten rather than calm an expectant mother's fears. And a resident's rigorous schedule can leave little time for the necessary rest.

If that were not enough, program directors and male residents do not always smile upon the pregnant female resident. Not too long ago, the director of one famous residency program bluntly said that he found it quite inconsiderate for a woman in training to get pregnant.

So the obstacles abound. But they do not diminish the joy of bringing a child into the world. Also, while bearing a child—not to mention raising it—interrupts a career, it can make a female obstetrician a more sensitive, more understanding and more effective doctor.

Simply finding the time to get pregnant presents problems for a resident. Be prepared to be on call for at least three cycles of ovulation. And by the time the fourth cycle rolls around, you will be so neurotic you probably won't ovulate at all.

When you finally do manage to become pregnant and need to pick a physician, compose a list, and ask the obstetrician at the top of it if he or she will accept professional courtesy. Proceed down the list until you find someone who does. I had an essentially normal delivery and stayed in the hospital for a day and a half. Even so, I owed almost $800 for the deductable on the hospital bill and the epidural—which had to be placed twice because the resident missed the first time. That was from a total bill of nearly $3,750 (in 1981).

Problems for the expectant resident begin to multiply as soon as you start putting on the pounds. And the pounds. And the pounds. Physicians as a rule tend to fall into the slightly overweight and slightly underexercised category. For residents in particular, there simply isn't the time to slip away regularly to exercise classes. I gained 68 pounds.

If it is true that a little bit of knowledge is dangerous, a lot of knowledge can be positively deadly. What I knew mortified me. I suffered, for example, from recurring nightmares of ectopic gestations—in both tubes—or of giving birth to children for whose syndromes names had yet to be invented. It didn't help when the first two conferences I attended after receiving the positive pregnancy test results were "A Summary of Ten Years of Stillbirths at LA County Hospital," and "Ambiguous Genitalia in the New-born." Both replete with full color kodachromes.

Nor did the experiences of my colleagues reassure me. One pregnant resident I knew was present on the ward—although fortunately not the primary physician—when a woman with no previous prenatal care delivered a Rubella infant. My friend, as well as residents and doctors from all corners of the hospital, had to be quarantined until they were determined not to have contracted the disease. The incident was terrifying, but it did subsequently lead to better enforcement of screening and vaccination procedures against Rubella for all hospital employees.

Nor was the rest of my friend's pregnancy uneventful. We spent every waking moment avoiding patients with spots (thank goodness AIDS had not yet been invented). When she finally delivered a nine pound boy by forceps, she wound up with a broken coccyx, a foley catheter because she could not void and a post-partum hemorrhage that required transfusion. It was all very encouraging.

Fears of physical complications are not the only problem. Superstition creeps in. I mixed my urine with Drano to see what sex the baby would be. I stood in front of the mirror to see if I was carrying the baby low or high.

Then there was the problem of going to Lamaze class incognito. I didn't want the other women to know I was an obstetrician. They would find it hard to accept the fact that although I was professionally trained to deliver babies I was as inexperienced as they were in giving birth. I wanted my husband to attend classes as well. He didn't see the point. He too believed that because I was an obstetrician I knew everything. I had to drag him to the sessions.

The reaction of my patients was equally amazing. Some refused to believe that their doctor was pregnant. They could not reconcile the image of the glowingly expectant mother with that of the imperturbable, all-knowing physician. I began to think some of my infertility patients were downright hostile. Other patients seemed weirdly oblivious. When I was eight and a half months pregnant and routinely began informing patients that another doctor would cover for me when I delivered, I had patients stare at me and say, "You're pregnant?"

Except for gaining weight, my pregnancy went well, so I continued to work full time until the day I delivered. Being a chief resident in gynecology got hectic. If three ectopic gestations came in I would do one with the intern, one with the first year resident and one with the second year resident. I found, however, that most pregnant women, operating around their protruding stomachs, can perform as well as any overweight male doctor.

They teach you a lot about pain in medical school, and more about relieving it. But they don't teach you how to endure it. I have no tolerance for pain and the hysterical fear it can induce. Deep breathing is fine, but when one is truly scared, as I was, medication is the only answer. With anaesthesia I survived, and the calm that enveloped me after delivery was remarkable. My child instantly became my universe and the pain once again seemed an experience that others undergo.

Bearing a child does make an obstetrician more empathetic. The banalities of heartburn, hemorrhoids and maternity clothes become topics of great interest and extended conversation. To this day I quote what I learned as an expectant mother—none of which was covered in medical school or residency.

But empathy can bring pain—a lesson I had to be retaught. After the birth of my second child, the first patient I delivered when I returned to work was the 26-year-old receptionist of a colleague. She delivered a Down's Syndrome child. I almost couldn't bear to tell her, and that night I think I cried as much as she did.

Overnight in the CCU

Scott May

Three hours of inpatient child psychotherapy, an hour of outpatient therapy, ward rounds, an administrative lunch meeting, a seminar on consultation/liaison work, an hour of supervision, a meeting with the pediatric endocrinologist about the abnormal thyroid levels in one of my kids on the ward, and finishing all of my progress notes for the week before 7:30 so I can meet my girlfriend, Marilyn, in time to make the guitar concert at 8:00.

Once again I had pulled off what seemed like an amazing balancing act of competing demands, so Marilyn and I could have some enjoyment on a Friday evening. All this on just five hours of sleep since I had been awakened suddenly at 5 a.m. with a sharp and persistent pain just below my left scapula (shoulder blade). Ah, there was Marilyn at 7:45 with a couple of burritos we could inhale on the way to the concert. Not bad, I thought to myself, just 15 minutes behind schedule. We got to the concert just as it was beginning, and I figured I would start unwinding from the week as I got into the concert. The piano duet preceding the jazz guitarist was a pleasant surprise, and I could feel myself begin to relax from the stresses of the week, except that the pain I had experienced early in the morning was becoming noticeable again. By the time the jazz guitarist got rolling I found my attention divided between his music and my body's perplexing scapular pain.

My mind vaguely connected the fact that I had in fact had this pain earlier in the week (though higher in the shoulder), while jogging after work. It had gone away as soon as I had stopped jogging and I figured it was just mild phrenic nerve stretching caused by really expanding my lungs and diaphram as I was running hard.

By the second guitar piece I was really working hard to stay with the music. Instead, my mind was beginning to actively assess my pain, which now included a pleuritic component (i.e., the pain worsened when I inhaled) as well as a deep-shifting muscular component. My casual differential diagnosis of muscle spasms, a viral syndrome with muscular aches or viral pleurisy, gave way to a much more active consideration of big-time problems when I inexplicably developed shakes, chills, and sweating. My pulse was running at 85, a bit fast, but steady. I had no cough or other signs of pulmonary (lung) process, yet I found it strangely difficult to breathe, as though there were a tight band around my lungs making it hard to expand my chest.

Marilyn, noticing my shaking, had leaned over and asked if I was doing all right. Always one for understatements, I said I would be okay in a little while. I wasn't really so sure that I would be all right since none of my symptoms made medical sense to me. This wasn't so surprising given my desire to deny the significance of my pain and my exhaustion at the time. I began wondering if all this wasn't some psychological issue that was dramatically erupting from my unconscious in a physical form, and that maybe I was making too much of it. I tried to convince myself that if I would just concentrate more on the music it would all pass—hum, not so different than the magical thinking of one of the hospitalized children I had seen earlier in the day.

By the third guitar piece it really hurt to breathe and I began to feel "ill." I knew I was just a few minutes away from the UCLA emergency room where I had been on call two days earlier, but I wondered what they could really do that I hadn't already thought about. Sure, they could order a chest X-ray, some blood work, take my vital signs, but nothing definitive would come of it. Besides, I had been looking foward to this concert all week.

My mind moved to a patient I had taken care of during my internship when the pain really began getting to me. He had developed a fistula (open channel) between his pancreas and the tissue around his lungs and had complained of intense chest pain. Because he was a habitual opiate abuser, my medical resident thought he was just manipulating to get us to prescribe some demerol or other opiates. I remembered doing a pleural tap, and sure enough there was fluid around his lungs, filled with amylase. Maybe I too had a fistula, my lungs really hurt. Marilyn was becoming equally distracted as my sweating and shakes worsened and tried again to get me to go to the emergency room to find out what was going on. I was still holding out. I didn't want to be just another complaining patient for an overworked intern, and no doubt I'd feel embarrassed when he'd find out I was also on the housestaff.

Marilyn became insistent as I began to moan out loud, and I no longer had the energy to resist. Still, what were they going to find in the emergency room, and did I want to know if they did find something? I could barely make out the guitarist's burning improvizations as we made our way to the parking lot. I knew I was feeling terrible when I asked her to drive my car. Five minutes later I was speaking to the triage nurse in the E.R. explaining that I had chest pain and was on the housestaff. I was hoping to expedite this ordeal and make it back to the concert before it concluded. Somewhat to my surprise, she stood up and walked me back to a medical examining room. My blood pressure was normal, but my pulse was now 120, I was sweating more profusely and felt awful.

Perhaps, as a way to bind my anxiety, or maybe as a reflex habit after 8 years of medical training, I kept trying to refine my differential diagnosis taking into account the migrating quality of my pain and my rapid pulse. While the intern was asking me about my symptoms, I was trying to restrict my history to the most relevant data. One of the E.R. nurses apologized for having to stick me numerous times as she was trying to draw blood and start an I.V. The intern had a friendly way, but he looked worried. He asked me to lie flat on the examining table so he could start my I.V. My body suddenly rebelled, and, in some deep way, I knew something was seriously wrong with my body. I lost all my color, as well as my blood pressure, and began vomiting from what felt like my solar plexus. I remained dimly aware of a quickened pace of those around me, along with a significantly slowed EKG. I felt the sharp stabbing pain in my wrist of someone trying to pierce my radial artery to get an arterial blood gas. I also heard someone say that they had to go for a femoral (groin) stick to get any blood since all my veins had collapsed when my blood pressure dropped out.

I was given a nitroglycerin tablet to place under my tongue. I was both hoping that it would work and relieve my pain and that it would not work, since if it did it would indicate that I was having coronary artery spasms and maybe a heart attack. I could vaguely make out the intern's voice as he was looking at my EKG and mentioning huge ST elevations on the heart tracing. For the first time I began to realize that my current situation might be more than just a painful experience, but instead potentially life ending. I thought of Arthur Ashe, the superb UCLA tennis star who had a heart attack at my same age, 34.

Yet as bad as I felt, I did not feel my body saying to me that I was going to "exit." I summoned some hope and bravado and told the nurse to try getting blood one more time from my arm before sticking me in the groin. By now the medical resident had made it over to my bed as my blood pressure came back up to 50 mm of mercury. With a little more blood in my head and a little less pain, my brain moved past its primitive survival level and once again I tried to figure out what was happening to my body. I remember thinking, "well, at least I had some real physical findings, and no one will think I'm a hypochondriac and no one will suggest that it was just an anxiety reaction." Ten minutes later I was feeling considerably more at ease, and though I still had plueritic pain, I could breathe without great effort. The medical resident brought over the EKG tracing and told me that either I had pericarditis (an inflammation of the heart sac) or that I had infarcted (destroyed, blocked) three walls of my heart. When I asked him what he was going to do at the end of his 12-hour E.R. shift, I think he felt more relieved than I did, since no one who has just infarcted three walls of their heart can speak, let alone ask a personal question.

I asked if my girlfriend could come in, and he asked me if I would come in, explaining that until the serial cardiac enzymes (a blood test that indicates heart muscle destruction) came back, he couldn't be absolutely sure that it wasn't a myocardial infarction. I could remember those long nights I had spent as an intern in the I.C.U. waiting for the cardiac enzymes to come back to let me know whether my patients had destroyed massive amounts of their heart muscle or were experiencing other causes for their chest pain. I hesitated to come in the hospital as a patient, partly seeing it as a blow to my dwindling sense of omnipotence, and partly thinking about how much expense and hassle it would involve. This medical resident would have done well in psychiatry. Instead of trying some authoritarian approach or trying to out-rank me (not easily done as I was a year past my residency), he asked me to help him out, explaining how bad it would look if I left and then developed further complications. We agreed on one night. Minutes later the medical admitting team was at my bedside and I was refining my no-frills medical history.

I was wheeled up to the CCU (Cornonary Care Unit) for monitoring and felt rather self-conscious since I frequently walk through the CCU corridors on my way to psychiatric emergencies. I couldn't decide how I felt being referred to as a 34-year-old child psychiatrist with chest pain/rule out M.I. (mycordial infarction).

Then came the real psychological crunch as I had to put on hospital pajamas, get my wrist identification band and had the ice-cold bedpan placed by my bed. I was entering patienthood and leaving behind my identity as an invincible, hard-working, in-control physician. Two more medical histories, one for the intern and a more detailed one for the medical student. I was still thinking about how much teaching I was going to try to do as I spoke with the medical student. We made a deal, I could watch the baseball playoffs on TV with the sound off and in return I would answer all his questions.

I liked the nurse assigned to me. She realized I was still struggling with making the transition between physicianhood and patienthood. She asked me about my work at UCLA and casually explained the CCU routine. They wanted to give me something for sleep, probably Dalmane, but I wanted to have all my brain cells working optimally and so decided to pass on sleep. In addition, it still hurt to breathe and I couldn't find a comfortable position to settle in. Below all this, I was still finding it difficult to give up control and allow someone else to take care of me. The nurse pointed out the call button by the bed. I knew it was going to be a long night, not unlike a busy night when I was on-call myself. I had to figure out how to occupy myself for the next seven hours, until the results from the cardiac enzymes began to come back and the attending physician in cardiology came by for morning rounds.

My next real dilemma occurred around five in the morning. The sharp, penetrating pleuritic pain wrenched me out of a groggy state as I re-experienced difficulty breathing. The scientist in me knew that it was a good idea to re-test the nitroglycerin to see if it relieved my pain, but it meant waking up the intern and I wanted to give him a chance to get some sleep. The pain continued to escalate, and after fifteen minutes I called the nurse who told me that the intern was in fact sleeping. After thirty minutes I called her again and she told me the intern was awake but was now in the shower. She ran an EKG tracing herself and I just tried to hang on as each breath felt like someone was sandblasting my lungs.

The intern came by around 6 a.m. and seemed genuinely upset that I had not wakened him to let him know about the pain returning. He told me that my first set of cardiac enzymes were normal, and that he was relieved to see that I had developed a fever and generalized aches. This meant that I probably had a viral syndrome, and as this was the most common cause for pericarditis, it supported that diagnosis which I much preferred over a myocardial infarction (heart attack). I had been pleased with myself for remembering that coxsackievirus and echovirus were the main two viral culprits associated with pericarditis. I figured that one of the kids I had hospitalized on the psychiatry service was getting even with me for keeping him in the hospital by giving me the virus and keeping me in the hospital.

I remember waiting for the attending cardiologist and the medical team to make rounds much as a gymnast waits for his score after his event. The cardiologist gave me my performance numbers on the cardiac enzymes and EKG and rated the degree of likelihood (98%) of having pericarditis versus some other disorder. He told me that I had a classic presentation of symptoms as well as classic EKG findings, except for the fact that it was hard to hear a pericardial friction rub with his stethoscope. In fact, he asked if I minded if he used my EKG tracing for teaching purposes since it so clearly demonstrated the difficulty of distinguishing between pericarditis and a myocardial infarction. I told him that it would be fine and then caught him off guard. I asked about the chances of my going backpacking in the Sierra Nevadas in a few days as I had been planning to do, just after I finished asking him how to determine if one is developing cardiac tamponade, a potentially fatal sequela to pericarditis. His response demonstrated that he knew more medicine than just cardiology, as he no doubt picked up on my effort to retain some semblance of invincibility after this painful and scary episode. He didn't tell me not to go, but instead asked me two simple questions. He wondered how I would feel if I had a recurrence of the same symptoms that brought me into the CCU while I was thirty miles from the closest vehicle and one hundred miles from the nearest hospital. I realized at that moment, my denial and omnipotence did have some limits.

Following my discussion with the cardiologist, I called my backpacking partner and several family members. They were funny phone calls, because in some way I was calling to say that I was returning to my role as doctor and leaving my role as patient, even though the people on the other end of the phone never knew I had left the role of doctor. I underlined this shift back to the doctor role when I stopped in the medical library and checked out eight journals (one on pericarditis) on my way out of the hospital, with the rationalization of not wanting to waste a trip to the hospital.

Arriving home left me with more time to myself to mull over the changes that I had gone through. I knew that I had a legitimate reason to take the week off, but did I want to? Was it fair to my patients who were all stuck in the hospital? Yet had it been my incessant working that had made me vulnerable to that damn coxsackievirus to begin with? Did I want to accept my vulnerability or go on pushing myself? Had I just been taught an important lesson relatively benignly or was it all just an unlucky accident? I compromised, and took off two days from work, and went easy the next three. I passed on the backpacking trip for a few weeks. I took some antiinflammatory medication for several days and gradually reassumed all one hundred percent of my role as a physician.

But I did not leave the CCU as the same person who had entered it. It's not something in my cardiac function that has changed, but rather in my psyche. When I walk past the CCU on my way to pediatrics or the emergency room it's not the same. I wrote a letter to the staff on the CCU and stopped by to thank several nurses there. I became friendly with one of the attending physicians and say hello to the CCU intern, who is now a resident, whenever I see him in the hospital. But the biggest change is knowing first hand the dependency and vulnerability that any patient feels when he or she comes into the hospital, regardless of what his or her previous role had been. I can feel so much more clearly the hopes and expectations that are directed toward the treating physician and realize that being a patient is just as difficult a role as it is to be a doctor. I also realized that I need to alter some of my own expectations of my role as a doctor if I want to make this experience a one-time visit to the CCU.

RECOMMENDED READING

Internship

Adler, Robert, Werner, Edwenna R., and Kursch, Barbara, 1980, "Systematic Study of Four Years of Internship," *Pediatrics*, Vol. 66, No. 6, pp. 1000–1008.

Boisaubin, Eugene V., 1981, "Reflections on Residency Training," *The Pharos*, Summer Issue, pp. 2–5.

Casscells, Ward, 1982, "Life (So to Speak) after Medical School," *Harvard Medical Alumni Bulletin*, Vol. 56, No. 1, pp. 22–24, 60.

Cassem, Edwin H., 1979, "Internship, Liberty, Death and Other Choices," *Harvard Medical Alumni Bulletin*, Vol. 53, No. 6, pp. 46–48.

Friedman, Richard C., Kornfeld, Donald S., and Bigger, Thomas J., 1973, "Psychological Problems Associated with Sleep Deprivation in Interns," *Journal of Medical Education*, Vol. 48, May Issue, pp. 436–441.

Reuban, David Bart, 1982, "The Intern's First Death: A Piece of My Mind," *Journal of the American Medical Association*, Vol. 248, No. 7, p. 821.

Schiedermayer, David L., 1983, "Drops of Blood: A Day in The Life of An Intern," *The New Physician*, No. 1, pp. 23–25.

Strasburger, Victor, 1981, "Internship: A Year Can Be a Very Long Time," *The New Physician*, Vol. 30, No. 2, pp. 26–27.

Turk, Emily R., 1984, "Matchmaking," *The New Physician*, Vol. 33, No. 3, pp. 17–18.

Valko, Robert J., and Clayton, Paula J., 1975, "Depression in The Internship," *Diseases of the Nervous System*, Vol. 36, No. 1, pp. 26–29.

Residency

Chamberlain, Allan, 1981, "Sleep Deprivation in Medical Education," *The New Physician*, Vol. 30, No. 4, pp. 28–30.

Gerritsen, Terry, 1984, "Thoughts of A Doctor Turned Mother," *The New Physician*, Vol. 33, No. 2, pp. 17–18.

Harwood, Michael, 1984, "The Ordeal: Life as a Medical Resident," *The New York Times Magazine*, June 3, 1984 Issue, pp. 39–45, 70–80.

Hunter, Thomas H., 1976, "How Many Hats Can a House Officer Wear?" *The New England Journal of Medicine*, Vol. 294, pp. 608–609.

Kielisch, Carl H., 1984, "Is It Worth It?—Hours versus Pay," *The Pre-Med Advisor*, April-May Issue, p. 7.

Krogh, Christopher, Vorhes, Carl, and Abbott, Geoff, "The Residency Interview: Advice from The Interviewers," *The New Physician*, Vol. 33, No. 5, pp. 8–12.

Loes, Michael W., and Scheiber, Stephen C., 1981, "The Impaired Resident: Psychiatric Disorders," *Arizona Medicine*, Vol. 38, No. 10, pp. 777–779.

Pfifferling, John-Henry, 1983, "Coping with Residency Distress," *Resident and Staff Physician*, Vol. 29, No. 10, pp. 105–111.

Yager, Joel, 1974, "A Survival Guide for Psychiatric Residents," *Archives of General Psychiatry*, Vol. 30.

3

Medical Practice
and Retirement

Medical training has been described as a prolonged state of adolescence. This is because financial, social, and emotional independence, the hallmark of adult maturity, usually eludes trainees until the completion of their residency training. In the medical center, close supervision is a way of life; relatively little trainee freedom exists for independent thought or action. But this changes precipitously when physicians finally leave the confines of the teaching hospital and venture forth into the community to make it on their own.

The prolonged training period required to become a specialized physician—four years of undergraduate work, four years of medical school, and two to seven years of residency training, depending upon the specialty—usually prolongs this adolescence-like period of dependence into the thirties. Then, upon entering medical practice, the physician is essentially told to "grow up."

Although the shift from dependence to independence may be eagerly anticipated, it is not always an easy transition. At age thirty, with financial, marital, and emotional debts to pay and many new challenges to confront, life can be complicated.

Unfortunately, little is said or done in medical school or postgraduate training to prepare physicians for this relatively uncharted course. Nor has much been written about the challenging psychosocial dilemmas that typically confront practicing physicians. Aside from romanticized television "soap operas," very little has been generated in the mass media about this developmental stage of the physician's personal and professional development. The earlier stages have captured the interest of the popular and scholarly media, but very little attention has been given to the early, middle, or senior years of medical practice. Largely unexplored are the personal struggles typically encountered after residency training.

A notable exception is the writing of McCue (1982), who catalogued some of the practical issues that typically confront physicians as they venture forth from the teaching hospital to make a living in the community. Immediate questions to be dealt with are: what type of practice to enter, how to find a job, how to evaluate a job offer, how to organize the finances and office, how to be an effective boss and manage personnel, how to set fees and collect them, how to organize medical records in a private practice, and how to organize time efficiently. These and many other issues must be braved by physicians who typically had had little, if any, formal training for such decisions.

Adjusting into the community may be especially difficult for physicians whose racial or ethnic background is distinct from the cultural milieu of the upper-middle class teaching hospital. For, as racial and ethnic minorities become socialized in the physician's career, they run the risk of becoming alienated from their communities of origin, even distrusted by their former associates. Families and former friends may find it difficult to understand the time demands made upon the physician. Because the professionalized demeanor and attitudes may be interpreted as interpersonal coldness and insensitivity, former associates may feel that the "uppity" doctor has left them behind. As such, the physician may feel caught between two worlds and experience difficulty in receiving much nurturance from either.

After extensively interviewing graduating resident physicians, Borus (1978) found that nearly all experienced anxiety and depression. Although they had looked forward to the day when they could finally make decisions as to what they would and would not do, when the time actually came it was not so easy. For one thing, they had to come face to face with their adolescent fantasy that physicians "can do anything and everything." Sudden confrontation between idealistic dreams and harsh realities can be discomforting. Facing the fact that one is unlikely to receive a Nobel Prize in Medicine or be chair of a prestigious medical school department may be difficult if one has held such grandiose fantasies about such achievements. To make the adjustment successfully, Borus counsels residents to realize that major changes are about to take place in their lives and that various considerations such as professional aspirations, per-

sonal needs, and family expectations must be thoughtfully priori-
tized.

Aside from these transition problems, practicing physicians also
experience many other sources of stress, some of which may have
been experienced during medical training. But now the full weight of
responsibility rests on them. The stressors that most typically occur
at this stage have been outlined by McCue (1982). Frequent
encounters with people who are in pain or otherwise uncomfortable
and unable to express gratitude can take a toll on the physician, as
does the need, with some procedures and therapies, of inflicting
pain and discomfort. The physician must also probe into intimate
histories and body parts which, in any other context, would be
considered highly inappropriate and deeply personal. The patient's
natural desire to preserve modesty and privacy often conflicts with
the physician's need to acquire clinical information.

Dealing with death can also be a constant threat, especially
when it is regarded as the physician's failure. Explaining to family
members that a loved one is dead or dying can be emotionally taxing.

Making clinical decisions on the basis of conflicting and/or
incomplete information is another source of stress, for such decisions
affect the health and welfare, even the lives, of patients. Unlike
earlier years, the practicing physician is less likely to have protective
mentors to fall back on.

On top of everything else, physicians must take care of what
James Groves (1978) calls "hateful patients." The first type of
troublesome patients are the *dependent clingers* who range from those
who make appropriate requests for reassurance to those who
repeatedly ask for explanations, affection, medications, and other
forms of attention. Second are *entitled demanders*, patients who use
intimidation, devaluation, and the induction of guilt to get what they
want. These patients try to control physicians by withholding
payment or other means. *Manipulative help-rejectors*, the third type,
create problems for physicians because no clinical regimen is seen by
them as effective in dealing with their medical problems. They keep
returning to their office to say that nothing works. *Self-destructive
deniers*, the final type, derive pleasure in undermining and defeating
the physician's attempt to help them. Daily encounters with such
patients do nothing to enhance the physician's state of emotional
well-being.

Such problems may be exacerbated when physicians are
stereotyped because of identifying characteristics such as age, skin
color, or physical handicap. When such physicians stand out as
different, it may be difficult to settle for just being good enough; they

must be better than others. Thus, a physician with a speech impediment, for example, may feel the pressure to be particularly brilliant when delivering the talk, just as elderly physicians cannot show difficulty when threading a catheter, as all do from time to time, or risk speculation about declined ability or senility.

Some patients may be less cooperative when the physician has a different skin color or other differing characteristic. Since effective treatment generally requires the patient's trust and cooperation, treatment effectiveness can be jeopardized. Such physicians have to overcome not just patients' medical problems, but also their prejudices.

Retirement is the most neglected and least frequently discussed of all the phases of physician development. This stage can be a time of loss, a period of declining productivity and self-worth. Such losses, of course, are not pleasant for anyone, but the discomfort might be particularly acute for physicians grown accustomed to considerable deference from others. Because few professions offer more status and respect, an erosion of patient deference may be a profound psychic loss.

As the practice of medicine shifts from small personalized offices of independent private practice to large medical corporations that employ physicians, the "pie" of financial profit is being divided into smaller pieces causing more and more physicians to be pushed out of private practice at earlier ages. Because medicine has traditionally been governed by conduct norms of "gentlemanliness," characterized by professional trust and good will, many retiring physicians have not protected themselves legally or otherwise from profit-oriented colleagues. The newer businesslike mentality, characterized by "cut-throat" competition, may come as a shock and result in a premature unwanted retirement.

Whether physician or some other professional, two essential requiremens are necessary for satisfactory retirement: health and a sufficient economic base. Fortunately, most physicians have enjoyed the economic rewards necessary for a comfortable retirement. But well-being may be jeopardized if years of demanding work schedules have led to a neglect of personal health.

The selections for this chapter provide further insight into these important issues. The first, "A Short Guide to Doctors," by John Secondi, is a tongue-in-cheek review of the old stereotypes about various medical specialists. A sampling of his written descriptions follow.

The General Practitioner, though nearly an extinct breed, is a warm, wonderful guy who always has time, the kind of person who knows patients inside and out from the moment of their delivery until his ink dries on their death certificates. The Internist is a general practitioner with more diplomas on the wall and without house calls. Pediatricians act and look like Peter Pan, wear saddle shoes and bow ties, are short, and never use words longer than two syllables or sentences of more than four words; a few skip during clinic. Plastic surgeons, gorgeous from every angle, wear expensive hand-tailored clothing and have sculptured features. Psychiatrists are easy to spot at cocktail parties because they either stare right at others or look through them, depending on which makes them feel more uncomfortable.

We have selected this article because it captures an insider's view of perceived physician idiosyncrasies. From the perspective of patients, who lack this insider's view, few differences separate one physician from another. Other than specialty designations, all doctors seem essentially alike. Once admitted to the inner sanctum of the physician's world, however, differences between specialists become readily apparent. For one thing, there is a good deal of competitive jockeying for status and professional recognition among physicians. Sometimes this takes the form of joking about other specialists. "Did you hear about the surgeon who holds the elevator door open with his head," the internist asks. "He thinks his hands are too valuable."

Laughter not only lightens the environment but also ventilates status resentments. In this case, the surgeon, who typically enjoys high prestige, is brought down to size. The joke also reinforces the hospital stereotype that surgeons are action-oriented rather than intellectual people who like to act but not think.

Interestingly, stereotypes about medical specialists often pertain to characteristics of the patients they serve. Thus, psychiatrists are characterized as a bit crazy, neurologists brainy, dermatologists superficial, and pediatricians child-like.

The next article, "Modern Times: The Business of Being a Doctor," by Sankey Williams, touches on a now-pervasive trend in medicine, the increasing concern about the business aspects of clinical practice. The author, a practicing physician, reflects on how the medical practice of his father differed from his own. In a much simpler day, Williams' father earned $25.00 per month as an intern, made housecalls, and had warm personal relationships with patients. Today's complicated system of health care, dominated by medical bureaucracies, presents a striking contrast unimaginable to those who practiced a few generations ago. Who would have anticipated such medical entities as HMOs (Health Maintenance

Organizations), PPOs (Preferred Providers Organizations) and DRGs (Diagnostic Related Groups)?

In a 20-year survey of articles in the *New England Journal of Medicine*, Klein and Small (1984) found that during the last two decades, the proportion of articles dealing with economic aspects of medical care increased nearly 400 percent. If this trend continues, they suggest changing the journal's name to "The New England Journal of Money and Medicine."

The third selection, "Facing Our Mistakes," by David Hilfiker, offers a rare glimpse of clinical failure, an infrequently acknowledged or discussed problem. One of the most difficult aspects for any physician is in coming to terms with medical mistakes. Because the practice of medicine is an art as well as a science, clinical decisions are often imprecise and faulty. The inevitable result is that, throughout a physician's lifetime, mistakes are bound to be made. Since medicine involves decisions that affect sickness and health, life and death, how does the physician cope with the knowledge of such mistakes? Hilfiker's open acknowledgement of a costly clinical error is an unusually courageous account that, in varying forms, could happen to any physician.

"The Doctor–Nurse Game," our fourth selection, was written two decades ago by Leonard Stein. Although times have obviously changed (for example, the doctors are not always "he" and the nurses "she"), basic elements of "the game" still persist and tend to follow the traditional male–female pattern. Even if the doctor is a woman and the nurse a man, the same power struggle (doctor = male role versus nurse = female role) may exist. Basically, the object of the game is the best treatment for the patient and mutual respect and cooperation between doctor and nurse. But the rules can be tricky. If the game is played correctly, both doctor and nurse (and patient) win; if not, all lose. The game is self-perpetuating, part of a set of attitudes and perceptions (the doctor's, the nurse's, and the general public's). It is a "transactional neurosis."

Stein's article makes clear that in any profession or business, there are formal and informal hierarchies, social pecking orders, and written and unwritten laws of conduct among professionals. But physicians and nurses are not the only ones who sometimes struggle to get along. There are chiropractors, osteopaths, physician's assistants, social workers, psychologists—and the list goes on. These health care practitioners often feel threatened by each other's expertise or drawing power. Competition is often a major bone of contention among them. Who will get the patients? Who will be considered the expert? Increasingly, less highly trained individuals provide some of the noncrucial care that physicians previously handled. And this can be frustrating to the physician. "I went to school for twelve years, slaved through internship and residency," a physician laments, "and now some physician's assistant comes right out of high school and a couple of years of training and is seeing *my* patients! It doesn't seem fair!"

Any discussion about the physician's experience is incomplete without considering the doctor's family life. The article by Robert Coombs, entitled "Structural Strain in the Medical Marriage," addresses this theme. Typically, each physician is involved in competing love affairs, one with a mate and the other with the career. And, as with any love triangle, it is not easy to achieve a compatible relationship between the two; each can profoundly affect the other.

By "structural strain" Coombs means those aspects of interpersonal strain between physician and spouse that typically occur, not because of personalities involved, but because the current system of medical training and practice fosters them. According to the author, all medical couples will experience some interpersonal strain due to absenteeism, status comparisons between the physician's spouse and others of the same sex, relative deprivation of the physician's status at home and at work, resistance in recognizing and seeking help with family problems, and the priority accorded to medical needs over family needs.

We conclude this chapter with an insightful article about retirement. In "A Physician's Prologue to Retirement," William J. Perry, M.D., tells about his own "phasing in" to retirement. In preparing for his semi-retirement Perry was forced to examine the feelings of status deprivation engendered by the loss of his practice. His sense of lost identity was profound. As soon as a physician makes the announcement to retire, he says, "you feel like an extra thumb in a five-finger glove." But satisfaction can be found in making up for past inequities in time and attention to one's family. Other satisfactions include shorter and less complicated workdays, vacations without monetary loss due to office absence, and the freedom to engage in mutually enjoyable activities with one's spouse. Although the adjustments are great, this period of life is not without its compensations, especially if health and a secure economic foundation have been carefully maintained.

REFERENCES

Borus, J. F., 1978, "The Transition to Practice," *American Journal of Psychiatry*, Vol. 135, pp. 1513–1516.

Groves, J. E., 1978, "Taking Care of the Hateful Patient," *The New England Journal of Medicine*, Vol. 298, pp. 883–887.

Klein, M. V., and Small, G. W., 1984, "Money and Medicine," *The New England Journal of Medicine*, Vol. 311, p. 542.

McCue, J. D., 1982, "The Effects of Stress on Physicians and Their Medical Practice," *The New England Journal of Medicine*, Vol. 306, pp. 458–463.

A Short Guide to Doctors

John J. Secondi

Medicine, like every other field these days, is so overspecialized that even a card-carrying doctor like me has trouble telling who's who. The layman, I imagine, is almost helpless to distinguish the forest from the tree surgeons. I have noticed, however, that my colleagues have a tendency to run to type. So, in an effort to clear up the confusion, I have compiled a little list so simple that the most naive patient can spot at a glance which doctor is which.

The General Practitioner: These gentlemen used to be the ones you saw most often, when you lived back in Nebraska and watched the cars go by from your front porch for entertainment. Now they are nearly extinct, like the buffalo and the stork, although there are a few left in a preserve in Iowa. Most of them looked like a cross between Charlie Ruggles and Colonel Sanders; they were warm, wonderful, and always had time for you, even if they slept only three hours a night. They knew you inside and out from the moment they delivered you until their ink dried on your death certificate, and they were always there to help you push your car out of the mud. If anybody knows where there's one of these left, please drop me a note. I could use a good doctor myself.

The Internist: This is a general practitioner with more diplomas on the walls and without house calls. (He also has money in the bank.) By the age of thirty at the latest he becomes obese, sallow, and emphysematous. Usually bald, he is always found sitting and smoking a pipe. (The pipe is a deliberate attempt to evoke the Delphic Oracle, which also simmered and steamed with ideas. The internist is nothing if not oracular.) As opposed to the surgeon, who carries no equipment at all except the keys to his Rolls Royce, the internist can be seen with a stethoscope protruding from one of thousands of pockets in his clothing. Really big stethoscopes are worn to give the impression of expertise in heart disease.

In his desk the internist stocks lifetime supplies of sample drugs; when you are in his office he may pick one or two at random and give them to you with alarming liberality. But don't worry; he won't let you know what they are. The internist is really happy only when deciding how to cope with some chronic incurable disease, preferably in a case some colleague has botched. The longer the name of the disease, the happier he is; and if it's in Latin he's ecstatic. An internist is required by law to have his phone ring twice an hour at least while he is at home, and he can never vacation. No internist's children ever become doctors.

The General Surgeon: These are the prima donnas of the trade. Today's surgeon is descended from the barbers of the Middle Ages, but washes more often. He may be fat or slim, but he is always loud, noticed, and in a hurry. He dashes dramatically in and out of rooms (whether patient, operating, or bath) and never lets you finish a sentence. To probing questions he nods wisely, smiles enigmatically, and runs off. (Never say "Now cut that out" to a surgeon.) He generally visits patients cloaked in green from head to toe to give the impression of being fresh from an operation, when probably (unless he is over fifty) he has been idling in his office all day waiting for someone—anyone—to call. After he does a surgical scrub, he raises his arms, which drip from the elbows. This posture serves both as a gesture to God for the usual assistance, and as a method to keep the bacteria flowing away from the surgeon—towards the patient.

Surgeons are taught early to rip off bandages as quickly as possible, pulling as much hair as they can get out with one clean tear. They have a distinctive jargon: For instance, they speak of healing by "primary intention" (which is to make lots of money), or by "secondary intention" (which means the wound got infected). If anything goes wrong during operations, surgeons are unanimous in blaming it on the anesthesiologists. Surgeons are the only doctors left who haven't cut out smoking, because they are confident they can cut out the cancer. If this description still doesn't make a surgeon flash in your mind, recall James Coburn in *Candy*. Absolutely accurate.

The Gastroenterologist: Gastrointestinal doctors, or "GI men," have had oral fixations since childhood. This means they are always talking a mile a minute, and at mealtimes they ingest like

Electroluxes. They're usually roly-poly, literary, and very pleasant to gossip with, as a consequence. The unsavoriness of their work is grossly exaggerated; nevertheless, they do receive a lot of cologne for Christmas. As kids they were the ones whose parents always had to bang on the bathroom door to get them out. If Alexander Woollcott had become a doctor, he would surely have been a gastroenterologist.

The Obstetrician-Gynecologist: The real wise guy in medicine. Sitting on their high stools day after day with their patients in that absurd saddle, these comedians see the funny side of life. They have to have a good sense of humor because otherwise they would be so nauseated by some of the things that come along they would swear off sex forever. Always ready with a wisecrack or a foul story (depending on whether you are a patient or another doctor), they are universally popular, except with pediatricians. Child doctors blame every childhood disease from thumb-sucking to Mongoloid idiocy on the anesthesia the obstetrician used. It is not true that all obstetrics is done at three o'clock in the morning. I personally recall one case in 1968 that was done at six in the morning, and others may have had similar experiences. Many Ob-Gyn men are now getting crash courses in abortion, which was never part of the medical curriculum before. These are the ones with sterile coathangers.

The Urologist: Urologists do for men what gynecologists do for women—more or less. They are drawn to their specialty irresistibly by its identification with the masses of tight curly hair they all have. Many urologists are now growing beards and muttonchops so you can spot them more easily than ever. Walking around weighted down by their waterproof rubber aprons and all those whiskers they resemble Noah before the flood. At home they putter around a lot with the kitchen sink to keep in practice. Like other plumbers they work good hours and make a good living.

The Anesthesiologist: Anesthesiology is the Tower of Babel of Medicine. There are a total of four English-speaking anesthesiologists in America: two on the East Coast, one in Chicago, and the other in L.A. All the others communicate with frenzied nasal accents or sign language. They are short, shy, retiring types who hide behind the sterile barrier during surgery and squeeze contentedly on their little black respiration bags. You will recall the bags from the 1930s movies because when Lionel Barrymore came too late they quit moving and you knew the patient had died.

The night before your next surgery an anesthesiologist may mince into you room, unheralded and uninvited. He will never show up after five o'clock, however. Without bothering to identify himself or even to ask for an intepreter, he will quiz you on all the allergies you may have. This is done to choose exactly the right toxin to put you to sleep with the next day; for God's sake, don't forget anything that might be relevant. Then he will bow graciously and back out of the room, and you'll never see him again. (Whether you'll see anyone else again is another question.) If you wake up from surgery, you may have a sore throat, even after an abdominal operation. This complication occurs because the anesthesiologist routinely puts the rubber airway down your esophagus six times before he finds the right hole. Anesthesiologists fear surgeons the way helpless children fear angry fathers. They are very sensitive and feel left-out enough, so be kind to them.

The Pediatrician: All pedi-pods, as they are called on the wards, act and look like Peter Pan. They wear saddle-shoes and bow ties, have cherubic faces, and wear crew cuts or pageboys, depending on whether they are over thirty. They are shorter than most other doctors, although they can be told from anesthesiologists because pediatricians are slightly taller, speak English, and have horizontally placed eyes. They never use words longer than two syllables or sentences of more than four words. Generally they sound as if they are doing Jonathan Winters imitations. Many have a lilting gait, and a few skip during clinic. About the age of forty they lose patience with all those frantic mothers and either commit suicide, go into research, or start child labor camps.

The Orthopedist: All bone doctors without exception are former college jocks or team managers; i.e., they are big brutes or mousy types who wish they were. They *all* wear white athletic socks. (This is the one infallible rule of medicine and makes it a snap to recognize an orthopedist.) They usually have plaster of paris splattered on their clumsy-looking shoes.

The Ophthalmologist: (This is the real "eye doctor" and is not to be confused with optometrists or opticians, who aren't M.D.'s at all.) Ophthalmologists, despite being constantly misspelled and mispronounced, are the happiest men in medicine. They work laughably few hours, make extravagant fees, and are adored by their patients, who understandably value their sight above all else. Thus ophthalmologists are always well-tanned and talk knowingly of Tahiti and the Riviera. They also play a great deal of golf. Curiously, they are uniformly tall, slim, and vaguely ethereal. A good example would be Pope Pius XII with a suntan. They use a jargon so technical and so infinitesimally detailed they cannot even make small-talk over drinks with other doctors.

The Otolaryngologist: When you've been to an ear, nose, and throat man you'll never forget it. These are the true sadists in medicine. Children despise them; they're the only doctors who make you feel worse than when you came in. What with the nausea produced by cocaine sprayed in the nose, and all those tiny little probes poking God-knows-where back in your sinuses, and all that blood swallowed after a tonsillectomy, going to an ENT man is like being used for an experiment by Edgar Allan Poe. The only common physical characteristic by which these gentlemen can be spotted is that they all still have their own tonsils.

The Plastic Surgeon: Immediately identifiable. They all wear hand-tailored clothing of vast expense and have sculptured features worthy of a Phidias or a Michelangelo. Gorgeous from every angle, they look years younger than they are, and boy do they know it. They were the big face men of college fraternities, the ones who were put strategically at the front door during rush week and in the first row in the yearbook picture. They are very rich because there are a lot of jealous women who will pay *anything* to look as good as the plastic surgeon. They have a tendency to get very snotty when you ask them what kind of plastic they're going to put in, and lecture you on the origin of the word "plastikos" in the traditions of Greek sculpture. Nevertheless, they have terrific guilt complexes about spending all their time on frivolous surgery, so they occasionally take on a burn victim to soothe their consciences. The patron saint of plastic surgery is Narcissus.

The Psychiatrist: Spotting a psychiatrist on the street is easy enough, but as he wanders on the wards of a state hospital he may need a nametag. Psychiatrists either avert their eyes from you or stare right through you, whichever makes you more uncomfortable. If they sense you're going to ask a question, they slip one in first. They never use complete sentences, only clauses and long words. I know a psychiatrist who begins every sentence with the word "that" and ends it with an exact quotation of Plato. The main object a shrink has in mind when he sees a patient is not to rescue the patient's sanity but to prove his. After all, how many surgeons do you know who have five years of operations on themselves before they can practice?

Today's psychiatric resident may have elbow-length hair, wear rings in one ear, and go to work in purple satin capes. This kind of psychiatrist has not hit Park Avenue yet, but it's only a matter of time. Incidentally, the reason there are so many Jewish psychiatrists is that they are basically yentas with M.D.'s.

The Radiologist: Radiologists hide in dark places and never come out, like other rodents. They make creepy-crawly gestures and rub their noses frequently. Their world is one of shadows and they detest the light of day. They hole up in leadened tunnels and, though they tell you that X-rays are harmless, they generally have their offspring as early as possible. (By the time they reach fifty irradiation has given their skins the texture of refried beans). Like Whistler, they view everyone as a study in black, white and gray. The thought of being responsible for a live human being is abhorrent to them. Yet they give off smiles of delicious perverse pleasure as they make patients swallow thick white slime and poke around in their bowels so their guts will show on film. Peter Lorre would have played a perfect radiologist.

I would like to complete the list, but I just got a frantic phone call from A.M.A. headquarters, and I have to run. Something about an emergency protest march against socialized medicine.

Modern Times:
The Business of Being a Doctor

Sankey V. Williams

My father had a lot to say about doctors and money, probably because he struggled with the issue all his life. Starting in a one-room school in eastern Kentucky, he received his M.D. from the University of Louisville in 1936. Throughout his undergraduate years during the Depression, he attended school one semester, and then worked the next so he could continue. I lost count of how many semesters he spent at which college.

His stories about the work were entertaining. As far as I know, it was the only time in his life he was shot at. In one of the state's poorer counties, where nearly everyone qualified for public assistance, he was at one time the clerk responsible for certifying need. One applicant disagreed with my father's assessment and took direct action. Luckily, he was a poor shot. Another job involved floating down the state's rivers identifying marijuana for destruction. It is easy to understand why these job alternatives did not keep him long from his childhood dream of becoming a doctor.

One of my father's favorite stories was about his first day as an intern. During a no-nonsense orientation, the sister in charge announced that the salary was $25 a month. Although room and board were provided, this sum was all he would have for personal expenses, which, as it turned out, included courting the pretty nurse who became my mother. He laughed when asked if each month's wages should be paid in cash or placed in a savings bond.

The economies of general practice in a small Kentucky town were clear, inescapable, and difficult. The rewards were not financial. My father loved his practice, and his patients were good to him in return. They treated him as an important and respected friend. Some of the children he delivered were named after him. There were other, more tangible, rewards. I remember the fresh tomatoes and corn brought to our back door at the end of the summer, and the baked goods and the occasional country ham during the holidays.

It was only later than I connected these gifts with the two filing cabinets in my father's office. Both contained large index cards on which he wrote a line or two along with the charge after each office visit. The filing cabinet of unpaid bills was almost full. The other was not. He would not turn away those who could not pay, and these were the people who brought their summer produce to our back door.

I never did figure out how much this arrangement bothered him. He took great pride in contributing his services to the community. But I remember mornings when he would return to join us for breakfast, exhausted after another late-night home delivery, with a full day's work in front of him. His pajamas would be sticking out from under his suit—there had been no time to dress properly when the call came. In telling the story, he had to mention that he had delivered six children to this family without payment, and his excitement was heightened by frustration and perhaps anger.

I also remember family talk about the county's other doctors. My father held them to a high standard, and often they did not measure up. This one did not pause to listen. That one meant well but had become outdated. Another had trouble understanding his patients because of a difference in cultural backgrounds. There was more sadness than disapproval in my father's voice—until he talked about their high fees. Worst were the outside doctors who sought his advice about opening a practice in this town that desperately needed more doctors: all they seemed interested in was the money.

Many may find all this hard to believe, but there was a time, not so far removed, when most doctors lived by the economic rules that determined my father's life. Some still do. For most of us, however, the options have changed. I am a general internist in a multispecialty group. Instead of index cards, we have a computer-based system that prints a "superbill" for third-party payers. As late as 1960, when my father's practice was most active, if health-care bills were paid, over half were paid directly by the patients themselves. In 1982, patients paid only 28 percent directly. (Government programs paid 47 percent, private insurance 29 percent.)

For my colleagues the question is not whether to provide care for those who will pay nothing, but whether to provide care for those whose third party will pay less than we charge. Our computer file of unpaid bills is much smaller than my father's file cabinet of never-to-be-paid bills, but that's not all that has changed. Our patients respect our skills and believe we are honest—but no one names children after us, and few bring us the fruit of their labor. I wonder how much this has to do with turning unpaid bills over to a collection agency, no matter how ethical, and how much is related to the monthly charts I receive from our business manager comparing my per-patient earnings with the group's mean.

My father was paid cash by the patient as the office visit was concluded, which forced both of them to consider the immediate value of the services rendered. I am paid a salary each month, plus an incentive based on "productivity."

The exchange of dollars is kept distant from me by my business office, and often from the patient by his or her third party. My patients and I use a modification of the fee-for-service system that shields both patient and doctor from the troubling business of deciding what medical care is worth, at least when the decision is made about how much care is needed. There is some value here, because the patient may not be prepared to make such an important decision when he or she is acutely ill, or is afraid that he or she might be.

How much such shielding has contributed to the increased cost of medical care is unknown, but some believe it is the principal cause. Certainly there are other causes. Every year I practice, there is more I can do that actually changes the outcome for more patients—new drugs, new diagnostic tests, new opportunities for referral to more specialized consultants, for still more unbelievable procedures. (It is sobering that my father's work was so valuable to his patients without these marvels of technology and science.) Although the benefit is worth the increased cost in these cases, the cost must be paid. Also, the number of elderly patients, and especially of "very elderly" patients, is growing, inevitably bringing greater cost because of their greater needs.

No matter how long the list of justifiable reasons for increased cost, however, it is true that some, perhaps most, costs could be reduced if greater effort were given to finding equally effective but less costly alternatives. How could it be otherwise under this payment system?

My practice operates under much the same fee-for-service system that my father's did. The more I do, especially the more procedures I perform, the more I am paid. When I am uncertain how much to do (and uncertainty seems to shadow every important decision), it is all too easy to do too much. My patient appreciates the effort; his or her third party does not complain about the price, as my patient might if he or she had to pay directly; and I can sleep better knowing that an extremely rare disorder has been eliminated from consideration in my diagnosis. To complete matters, my business manager calls to congratulate me for having raised my per-patient earnings above the mean.

When Steve Schroeder '64, pioneer investigator in this field, examined this issue several years ago in the journal *Medical Care*, he concluded that doctors could triple their office income by spending less time talking with patients and thinking about their problems, and more time performing diagnostic tests and other procedures.

It is for this reason that those who are most concerned about cost are supporting alternative payment systems for doctors. Some of the alternatives have been around so long that they are generally accepted, such as the straight salary system. Others, like the health maintenance organization (HMO), and the independent practice association (IPA), have become so common in recent years that they no longer seem strange.

In HMOs and IPAs, the group's income depends on the difference between the patients' predetermined capitation fee and the cost of care, which puts the HMOs or IPA at risk for real losses if too much is done at too high a cost. Years of study have shown that HMOs and IPAs do have lower costs, by as much as 10 to 40 percent, and that there are few differences in the type of care that is provided, except that patients are admitted to the hospital less often.

What remains unclear, however, is why this reduction occurs. It may result from the clinical styles of the doctors who choose this type of practice, from the better health of the people who join, from the economies of scale and more intensive peer review that are inherent to these large organizations, or from the improved management provided by the professional administrators. It is unclear what role the doctor's financial stake plays, in part because there are so many different payment arrangements, ranging from straight salary to direct risk sharing.

Many observers believe that HMOs and IPAs, regardless of their effectiveness, will not solve the problem of rising costs, because not everyone likes being restricted to a single HMO's doctors and sites. Optimistic estimates are that only 20 percent of the population will join, even when HMOs and IPAs become much more widespread than they are now.

Newer arrangements (with obligatory three-letter acronyms) have therefore been developed. They include the Diagnosis Related Group (DRG) system and the preferred provider organization (PPO). If my group were to become a PPO, it would contract with a third-party payer to provide services for reduced fees. In return, the third-party payer would waive some of its deductible and copayment requirements when subscribers came to us, which would encourage them to use us instead of someone else.

Theoretically, everyone would benefit. The total medical bill would be lower because of our reduced fees; my group would more than make up for the lower fees by seeing more patients; subscribers would have freedom of choice, yet many would pay less out of pocket; and the third party would attract more subscribers. Although other doctors would lose their patients to us, they could start their own PPO—and increased competition is the ultimate goal anyway.

California and some other states have begun experimenting with PPOs, but too little is known yet about whether they control costs or cause new problems. I wonder about the preservation of the fee-for-service incentive. Once every doctor has become a member of a PPO, everyone's fees will be lower. Still, all of us will be paid more when we do more to each patient, and we may be tempted to do too much, as greater competition will prevent us from raising prices to maintain our incomes.

The DRG system may offer a viable alternative. Based on the perceived success of a statewide demonstration project in New Jersey, the Health Care Financing Administration has begun paying acute-care general hospitals for Medicare patients under the DRG system in 46 states. No matter how long the patient stays, or how much the care costs, the hospital is paid a standard amount that depends on the patient's case type.

Case types are defined using several characteristics, including the patient's diagnoses, age, and surgical procedures. Each case type forms a separate "diagnosis related group," or DRG. Because payment does not depend on cost, the hospital loses money when costs are greater than the standard amount, and profits when they are less.

The DRG system puts powerful incentives in place: the hospital's very survival may depend on its ability to control costs. To control the unit cost of each service, the hospital must bargain more effectively with employees, and it must seek less expensive sources of supplies and equipment. To respond most effectively, the hospital also must find some way to reduce the number, and change the mix, of services provided to its patients—without changing the outcomes. Because the hospital's doctors order all these services, the hospital must, therefore, find some way to influence clinical practice.

Although this hospital focus on clinicians is reason enough for doctors to be interested in the DRG concept, there is more. If successful for the payment of hospitals, the DRG system likely will be extended to the payment of doctors. Most observers predict that the system will be successful, although no convincing evidence is yet available. This perception is so strong that some Blue Cross organizations already have adopted the DRG system for their patients' hospital payments. To prepare for the possibility of a prospective payment system for doctors, Congress has instructed the Health Care Financing Administration to design a system by October 1985.

It is unclear how such a system might work. In the mid-1970s Pennsylvania Blue Shield conducted a pilot study that could serve as an example. Ninety-one doctors in 10 hospitals agreed to receive a single, lump-sum payment for their services when patients with one of 23 selected diagnoses were admitted to the hospital—regardless of how long the patients stayed or how many services were provided.

The lump-sum payment was calculated as the average amount paid for physician services for that diagnosis in the previous year, adjusted for inflation. Using historical and concurrent controls, the patients in the study group had lengths of stay three percent shorter, and costs close to one percent lower, considering hospital and physician costs together. While small, these differences were statistically significant.

I can only speculate about what my father would say regarding all this. Probably he would wonder why we are spending so much energy worrying about getting paid when so much real doctoring remains to be done. This was one response he had to the turmoil that preceded the introduction of Medicare and Medicaid in 1966, although conservative politics influenced his position (which I disagreed with then because I mistakenly thought that I knew enough to do so).

In my father's time and place, the question of payment was no less real and no less important. There was, however, a clearer understanding about what a doctor should strive for when providing care and asking for payment.

Today we know better how to run the business of being a doctor, or we band together in groups and hire someone to do it for us. We also know how to make more accurate diagnoses, cure more people, and relieve more physical suffering. We cannot, however, improve on the respect and understanding that once passed between some country doctors and their patients. Our future would be more satisfying if we tried harder to recapture those relationships as we design the grand schemes that might lead to lost control.

Facing Our Mistakes

David Hilfiker

Looking at the appointment book for July 12, 1978, I notice that Barb Daily will be in today for her first prenatal examination. "Wonderful," I think, remembering my joy as I helped her deliver her first child two years ago. Barb and her husband Russ are friends, and our relationship became much closer with the shared experience of that birth. With so much exposure to disease every day in my rural family practice, I look forward to today's appointment with Barb and to the continuing relationship over the next months.

Barb seems to be in good health with all the symptoms and signs of pregnancy, but her urine pregnancy test is negative. I reassure Barb and myself that she is fine and that the test just hasn't turned positive yet. Rescheduling another test for the following week, I congratulate her on her condition and promise to get all her test results to her promptly.

But the next urine test is negative, too, which leaves me troubled. Isn't Barb pregnant? Has she had a missed abortion? I could make sure right now, of course, by ordering an ultrasound, but the new examination is available only in Duluth, 110 miles away from our northern Minnesota village, and it is expensive. I am aware of the Dailys' modest income. Besides, by waiting a few weeks, I'll find out for sure without the ultrasound. I call Barb on the phone and tell her about the negative test, about the possible abortion, and about the necessity of a repeat appointment in a few weeks if her next menstrual period does not occur on schedule.

It is, as usual, a hectic summer, and I almost forget about Barb's situation until a month later when she returns. Still no menstrual period, no abortion. She is confused and upset, since, she says, "I feel so pregnant." I am bothered, too, especially because her uterus continues to be enlarged. Her urine test remains definitely negative.

I break the bad news to her. "I think you have a missed abortion. You were probably pregnant, but the baby appears to have died some weeks ago, before your first examination. Unfortunately, you didn't have the miscarriage to get rid of the dead tissue from the baby and the placenta. If a miscarriage does not occur within a few weeks, I'd recommend a reexamination, another pregnancy test, and if nothing shows up, a dilation and curettage to clean out the uterus."

Barb is disappointed and saddened; there are tears. Both she and Russ have sufficient background in science to understand the technical aspects of the situation, but that doesn't alleviate the sorrow. We talk in the office at some length and make an appointment for two weeks later.

When Barb returns, Russ is with her. Still no menstrual period, no miscarriage, and a negative pregnancy test. It is difficult, but it also feels right to be able to share in friends' sadness. Thoroughly reviewing the situation with both of them, I schedule the D and C for later in the week.

Friday morning, when Barb is wheeled into the operating room, we chat before she is put to sleep. The surgical nurses in our small hospital are all friends, too, so the atmosphere is warm and relaxed. After induction of anesthesia, I examine Barb's pelvis. To my hands, the uterus now seems bigger than it had two days previously, but since all the pregnancy tests were negative, the uterus couldn't have grown. I continue the operation.

But this morning there is considerably more blood than usual, and it is only with great difficulty that I am able to extract any tissue. The body parts I remove are much larger than I had expected, considering when the fetus died, and they are not the decomposing tissue I'd anticipated. These are body parts that were recently alive! I suppress the rising panic in my body and try to complete the procedure. I am unable to evacuate the uterus completely, however, and after much sweat and worry, I stop, hoping that the uterus will expel the rest within a few days.

Russ is waiting outside the operating room, so I sit with him for a few minutes, telling him that Barb is fine but that there were some problems with the procedure. Since I haven't completely thought through what has happened, I can't be very helpful in answering his questions. I leave hurriedly for the office, promising to return that afternoon to talk with them once Barb has recovered from the anesthesia.

In between seeing other patients in the office that morning, I make several rushed phone calls, trying to figure out what has happened. Despite reassurances from the pathologist that it is statistically "impossible" for four consecutive pregnancy tests to be negative during a viable pregnancy, the horrifying awareness is growing that I have probably aborted Barb's living child. I won't know for sure until several days later, when the pathology report is available. In a daze I walk over to the hospital and try to tell Russ and Barb as much as I know, without telling them all that I suspect. I tell them that there may be more tissue expelled and that I won't know for sure about the pregnancy until the next week.

I can't really face my own suspicions yet.

That weekend I receive a tearful call from Barb. She has just passed some recognizable body parts of the baby; what is she to do? The bleeding has stopped, and she feels physically well, so it is apparent that the abortion I began on Friday is now over. I schedule a time in midweek to meet with them and review the entire situation.

The pathology report confirms my worst fears: I have aborted a living fetus at about 13 weeks of age. No explanation can be found for the negative pregnancy tests. My consultation with Barb and Russ later in the week is one of the hardest things I have ever done. Fortunately, their scientific sophistication allows me to describe in some detail what I have done and what my rationale was. But nothing can obscure the hard reality: I have killed their baby.

Politely, almost meekly, Russ asks whether the ultrasound examination could not have helped us. It almost seems that he is trying to protect my feelings, trying to absolve me of some of the responsibility. "Yes," I answer, "if I had ordered the ultrasound, we would have known that the baby was alive." I cannot explain to him why I didn't recommend it.

Over the next days and weeks and months, my guilt and anger grow. I discuss the events with my partners, with our pathologist, and with obstetric specialists. Some of my mistakes are obvious: I relied too heavily on one particular test; I was not skillful in determining the size of the uterus by pelvic examination; I should have ordered the ultrasound before proceeding with the D and C. Other mistakes become apparent as we review my handling of the case. There is simply no way I can justify what I have done. To make matters worse, complications after the D and C have caused much discomfort, worry, and expense. Barb is unable to become pregnant again for two years.

As physicians our automatic response to reading about such a tragedy is to try to discover what went wrong, to analyze why the mistakes occurred, and to institute corrective measures so that such things do not happen again. This response is important, indeed necessary, and I spent hours in such a review. But it is inadequate if it does not address our own emotional and spiritual experience of the events.

Although I was as honest with the Dailys as I could be in those next months, although I told them everything they wanted to know and described to them as completely as I could what had happened, I never shared with them the agony that I underwent trying to deal with the reality of the events. I never did ask for their forgiveness. I felt somehow that they had enough sorrow without having to bear my burden as well. Somehow, I felt, it was my responsibility to deal with my guilt alone.

Everyone, of course, makes mistakes, and no one enjoys the consequences. But the potential consequences of our medical mistakes are so overwhelming that it is almost impossible for practicing physicians to deal with their errors in a psychologically healthy fashion. Most people—doctors and patients alike—harbor deep within themselves the expectation that the physician will be perfect. No one seems prepared to accept the simple fact of life that physicians, like anyone else, will make mistakes.

By the very nature of our work, we physicians daily make decisions of extreme gravity. Our work in the intensive-care unit, in the emergency room, in the surgery suite, or in the delivery room offers us hundreds of opportunities daily to miscalculate, often with drastic consequences.

And it is not only in these settings but also in the humdrum of routine daily care that a physician can blunder into tragedy. One evening, for instance, a local boy was brought to the emergency room after an apparently minor automobile accident. One leg and foot were injured, but he was otherwise fine. After examining him, I consulted by telephone with an orthopedic surgeon in Duluth, and we decided that I would try to correct what appeared on the X-ray film to be a dislocated foot. As usual, I offered the patient and his mother (who happened to be a nurse with whom I worked regularly) a choice: I could reduce the dislocation in our small hospital or they could travel to Duluth to see the specialist. I was somewhat offended when they decided they would go to Duluth. My feelings changed considerably when the surgeon called me the next morning to thank me for the referral. He reported that the patient had not had a dislocation at all but a severe posterior compartment syndrome, which had hyperflexed the foot, causing it to appear dislocated. The posterior compartment had required immediate surgery the previous night in order to save the muscles of the lower leg. I felt physically weak as I realized that this young man would have been permanently injured had his mother not decided on her own to take him to Duluth.

Although much less drastic than the threat of death or severe disability, perhaps the most frequent result of physician misjudgment is the wasting of money, often in large amounts. Every practicing physician spends thousands of dollars of patients' money every day in the costs for visits, laboratory examinations, medications, and hospitalizations. An unneeded examination, the needless admission of a patient to the hospital, even the unnecessary advice to stay home from work can waste large amounts of money— frequently, the money of people who have little to spare. One comes to feel that any decision may have important consequences.

The cumulative impact of such mistakes (and the ever-present potential for many others) has had a devastating effect on my own emotional health, as it does, I believe, for most physicians. For it is not only the obvious mistakes with obvious results that trouble us. Such mistakes as I made with Barb are fortunately rare occurrences for any physician, and an emotionally mature person may learn to cope with them. But there are also those frequent times when an obvious mistake may lead to less obvious consequences, when the physician errs in judgment, never to know how important the error was.

Some years ago, as I was rushing to an imminent delivery, a young woman stopped me in the hospital hall to tell me that her mother had been having chest pains all night. Should she be brought to the emergency room? I knew her mother well, had examined her the previous week, and knew of her recurring angina. "No," I responded, thinking primarily of my busy schedule and the fact that I was already an hour late because of the unexpected delivery. "Take her over to the office, and I'll see her there as soon as I'm done here." It would be a lot more convenient to see her in the office, I thought. About 20 minutes later, as I was finishing the delivery, our clinic nurse rushed into the delivery room, her face pale and frantic. "Come quick! Mrs. Martin just collapsed." I sprinted the 100 yards to the office to find Mrs. Martin in cardiac arrest. Like many physician offices at that time, ours was not equipped with the advanced life-support equipment necessary to handle the situation. Despite everything we could do, Mrs. Martin died.

Would she have survived if I had initially agreed to see her in the emergency room where the requisite staff and equipment were available? No one will ever know for sure, but I have to live with the possibility that she might have lived if I had made a routine decision differently, a decision similar to many others I would make that day, yet one with such an overwhelming outcome.

There is also the common situation of the seriously ill, hospitalized patient who requires almost continuous decision making on the part of the physician. Although no "mistake" may be evident, there are always things that could have been done better: a little more of this medication, starting that treatment a little earlier, recognizing this complication a bit sooner, limiting the number of visitors, and so forth. If the patient dies, the physician is left wondering whether the care provided was adequate. There is no way to be certain, for no one can know what would have happened if things had been done differently. Usually, in fact, it is difficult to get an honest opinion from consultants and other physicians about what one could have done differently. (Judge not, that you not be judged?) In the end, the physician has to swallow the concern, suppress the guilt, and move on to the next patient. He or she may simply be unable to discover whether the mistakes were responsible for the patient's death.

Worst of all, the possibility of a serious mistake is present with each patient the physician sees. The inherent uncertainty of medical practice creates a situation in which errors are always possible. Was that baby I just sent home with a diagnosis of a mild viral fever actually in the early stages of a serious meningitis? Could that nine-year-old with stomach cramps whose mother I just lectured about psychosomatic illness come in to the hospital tomorrow with a ruptured appendix? Indeed, the closest I have ever come to involvement in a courtroom malpractive case was the result of my treatment of an apparently minor wrist injury one week after it happened: I misread a straightforward X-ray film and sent the young boy home with a diagnosis of sprain. I next heard about it five years later, when after being summoned to a hearing, I discovered that the fracture I had missed had not healed, and the patient had required extensive treatment and difficult surgery years later.

As practicing primary-care physicians, then, we work in an impossible situation. Each of the myriad decisions to be made every day has the potential for drastic consequences if it is not determined properly. And it is highly likely that sooner or later we will make the mistake that kills or seriously injures another person. How can we live with that knowledge? And after a serious mistake has been made, how can we continue in daily practice and expose ourselves again? How can we who see ourselves as healers deal with such guilt?

Painfully, almost unbelievably, we physicians are even less prepared to deal with our mistakes than the average lay person is. The climate of medical school and residency training, for instance, makes it nearly impossible to confront the emotional consequences of mistakes; it is an environment in which precision seems to predominate. In the large centers where doctors are trained, teams of physicians discuss the smallest details of cases; teaching is usually conducted to make it seem "obvious" what decisions should have been made. And when a physician does make an important mistake, it is first whispered about in the halls, as if it were a sin. Much later, a case conference is called in which experts who have had weeks to think about the situation discuss the way it should have been handled. The environment in which physicians are trained does not encourage them to talk about their mistakes or about their emotional responses to them.

Indeed, errors are rarely admitted or discussed once a physician is in private practice. I have some indication from consultants and colleagues that I am of at least average competence as a physician. The mistakes I have discussed here represent only a fraction of those of which I am aware. I assume that my colleagues at my own clinic and elsewhere are responsible for similar numbers of major and minor errors. Yet we rarely discuss them; I cannot remember a single instance in which another physician initiated a discussion of a mistake for the purpose of clarifying his or her own emotional response or deciding how to follow up. (I do not wish to imply that we don't discuss difficult cases or unfortunate results; yet these discussions are always handled so delicately in the presence of the "offending" physician that there is simply no space for confession or absolution.)

The medical profession simply seems to have no place for its mistakes. There is no permission given to talk about errors, no way of venting emotional responses. Indeed, one would almost think that mistakes are in the same category as sins: it is permissible to talk about them only when they happen to other people.

If the profession has no room for its mistakes, society seems to have even more rigid expectations of its physicians. The malpractice situation in our country is symptomatic of this attitude. In what other profession are practitioners regularly sued for hundreds of thousands of dollars because of a misjudgment? A lawyer informed me I could be sued for $50,000 for misreading the X-ray film that led to the young man's unhealed fracture. I am sure the Dailys could have successfully sued me for large amounts of money, had they chosen to do so. Experienced physicians who are honest with themselves can count many potential malpractice suits against them. Even the word "malpractice" carries the implication that one has done something more than make a natural mistake; it connotes guilt and sinfulness.

It is easy, of course, to understand why this situation has arisen. These mistakes are terrible; their consequences are drastic; and the victim or family should be compensated for medical bills, time lost from work, and suffering or death. But in our society, rather than establish a "patient compensation fund" (similar to worker's compensation) from which a deserving patient can be compensated for an injury that results from a legitimate mistake, we insist that the doctor be sued for "malpractice," judged guilty, and forced to compensate the patient personally. An atmosphere of denial is created: the "good physician" doesn't make mistakes.

The drastic consequences of our mistakes, the repeated opportunities to make them, the uncertainty about our own culpability when results are poor, and the medical and societal denial that mistakes must happen all result in an intolerable paradox for the physician. We see the horror of our own mistakes, yet we are given no permission to deal with their enormous emotional impact; instead, we are forced to continue the routine of repeatedly making decisions, any one of which could lead us back into the same pit.

Perhaps the only adequate avenue for dealing with this paradox is spiritual. Although mistakes are not usually sins, they engender similar feelings of guilt. How can I not feel guilty about the death of Barb's baby, the lack of adequate emergency care for Mrs. Martin, the fracture that didn't heal? Whether I "ought" to feel guilty is a moot point; most of us do feel guilty under such circumstances.

The only real answer for guilt is spiritual confession, restitution, and absolution. Yet within the structure of modern medicine there is simply no place for this spiritual healing. Although the emotionally mature physician may find it possible to give the patient or family a clinical description of what happened, the technical details are often so difficult for the lay person to understand that the nature of the mistake is hidden. Or if an error is clearly described, it is presented as "natural," "understandable," or "unavoidable" (which, indeed, it often is). But there is no place for real confession: "This is the mistake I made; I'm sorry." How can one say that to a grieving mother, to a family that has lost a member? It simply doesn't fit into the physician–patient relationship.

Even if one were bold enough to consider such a confession, strong voices would raise objections. When I finally heard about the unhealed fracture in my young patient, I was anxious that the incident not create antagonism between me and the family, since we live in a small town and see each other frequently. I was tempted to call the family and express my apologies and the hope that a satisfactory settlement could be worked out. I mentioned that possibility to a malpractice lawyer, but he was strongly opposed, urging me not to have any contact with the family until a settlement was reached. Even if a malpractice suit is not likely, the nature of the physician–patient relationship makes such a reversal of roles "unseemly." Can I further burden an already grieving family with the complexities of my feelings, my burden?

And if confession is difficult, what are we to say about restitution? The very nature of our work means that we are dealing with elements that cannot be restored in any meaningful way. What can I offer the Dailys in restitution?

I have not been successful in dealing with the paradox. Any patient encounter can dump me back into the situation of having caused more harm than good, yet my role is to be a healer. Since there has been no permission to address the paradox openly, I lapse into neurotic behavior to deal with my anxiety and guilt. Little wonder that physicians are accused of having a God complex; little wonder that we are defensive about our judgments; little wonder that we blame the patient or the previous physician when things go wrong, that we yell at the nurses for their mistakes, that we have such high rates of alcoholism, drug addiction, and suicide.

At some point we must bring our mistakes out of the closet. We need to give ourselves permission to recognize our errors and their consequences. We need to find healthy ways to deal with our emotional responses to those errors. Our profession is difficult enough without our having to wear the yoke of perfection.

The Doctor–Nurse Game

Leonard I. Stein

The relationship between the doctor and the nurse is a very special one. There are few professions where the degree of mutual respect and cooperation between co-workers is as intense as that between the doctor and nurse. Superficially, the stereotype of this relationship has been dramatized in many novels and television serials. When, however, it is observed carefully in an interactional framework, the relationship takes on a new dimension and has a special quality which fits a game model. The underlying attitudes which demand that this game be played are unfortunate. These attitudes create serious obstacles in the path of meaningful communications between the physicians and nonmedical professional groups.

The physician traditionally and appropriately has total responsibility for making the decisions regarding the management of his patients' treatment. To guide his decisions he considers data gleaned from several sources. He acquires a complete medical history, performs a thorough physical examination, interprets laboratory findings, and at times, obtains recommendations from physician-consultants. Another important factor in his decision-making are the recommendations he receives from the nurse. The interaction between doctor and nurse through which these recommendations are communicated and received is unique and interesting.

THE GAME

One rarely hears a nurse say, "Doctor I would recommend that you order a retention enema for Mrs. Brown." A physician, upon hearing a recommendation of that nature, would gape in amazement at the effrontery of the nurse. The nurse, upon hearing the statement, would look over her shoulder to see who said it, hardly believing the words actually came from her own mouth. Nevertheless, if one observes closely, nurses make recommendations of more import every hour and physicians willingly and respectfully consider them. If the nurse is to make a suggestion without appearing insolent and the doctor is to seriously consider that suggestion, their interaction must not violate the rules of the game.

Object of the Game

The object of the game is as follows: the nurse is to be bold, have initiative, and be responsible for making significant recommendations, while at the same time she must appear passive. This must be done in such a manner so as to make her recommendations appear to be initiated by the physician.

Both participants must be acutely sensitive to each other's nonverbal and cryptic verbal communications. A slight lowering of the head, a minor shifting of position in the chair, or a seemingly nonrelevant comment concerning an event which occurred eight months ago must be interpreted as a powerful message. The game requires the nimbleness of a high wire acrobat, and if either participant slips the game can be shattered; the penalties for frequent failure are apt to be severe.

Rules of the Game

The cardinal rule of the game is that open disagreement between the players must be avoided at all costs. Thus, the nurse must communicate her recommendations without appearing to be making a recommendation statement. The physician, in requesting a recommendation from a nurse, must do so without appearing to be asking for it. Utilization of this technique keeps anyone from committing themselves to a position before a sub rosa agreement on that position has already been established. In that way open disagreement is avoided. The greater the significance of the recommendation, the more subtly the game must be played.

To convey a subtle example of the game with all its nuances would require the talents of a literary artist. Lacking these talents, let me give you the following example which is unsubtle, but happens frequently. The medical resident on hospital call is awakened by telephone at 1 a.m. because a patient on a ward, not his own, has not been able to fall asleep. Dr. Jones answers the telephone and the dialogue goes like this:

> This is Dr. Jones.
> (An open and direct communication.)
> Dr. Jones, this is Miss Smith on 2 W—Mrs. Brown, who learned today of her father's death, is unable to fall asleep.
> (This message has two levels. Openly, it describes a set of circumstances, a woman who is unable to sleep and who that morning received word of her father's death. Less openly, but just as directly, it is a diagnostic and recommendation statement; i.e., Mrs. Brown is unable to sleep because of her grief, and she should be given a sedative. Dr. Jones, accepting the diagnostic statement and replying to the recommendation statement, answers.)
> What sleeping medication has been helpful to Mrs. Brown in the past?
> (Dr. Jones, not knowing the patient, is asking for a recommendation from the nurse, who does know the patient, about what sleeping medication should be prescribed. Note, however, his question does not appear to be asking her for a recommendation. Miss Smith replies.)
> Pentobarbital mg 100 was quite effective night before last.
> (A disguised recommendation statement. Dr. Jones replies with a note of authority in his voice.)
> Pentobarbital mg 100 before bedtime as needed for sleep, got it?
> (Miss Smith ends the conversation with the tone of a grateful supplicant.)
> Yes I have, and thank you very much doctor.

The above is an example of a successfully played doctor–nurse game. The nurse made appropriate recommendations which were accepted by the physician and were helpful to the patient. The game was successful because the cardinal rule was not violated. The nurse was able to make her recommendation without appearing to, and the physician was able to ask for recommendations without conspicuously asking for them.

The Scoring System

Inherent in any game are penalties and rewards for the players. In game theory, the doctor–nurse game fits the nonzero sum game model. It is not like chess, where the players compete with each other and whatever one player loses the other wins. Rather, it is the kind of game in which the rewards and punishments are shared by both players. If they play the game successfully they both win rewards, and if they are unskilled and the game is played badly, they both suffer the penalty.

The most obvious reward from the well-played game is a doctor–nurse team that operates efficiently. The physician is able to utilize the nurse as a valuable consultant, and the nurse gains self-esteem and professional satisfaction from her job. The less obvious rewards are no less important. A successful game creates a doctor–nurse alliance; through this alliance the physician gains the respect and admiration of the nursing service. He can be confident that his nursing staff will smooth the path for getting his work done. His charts will be organized and waiting from him when he arrives, the ruffled feathers of patients and relatives will have been smoothed down, his pet routines will be happily followed, and he will be helped in a thousand and one other ways.

The doctor–nurse alliance sheds its light on the nurse as well. She gains a reputation for being a "damn good nurse." She is respected by everyone and appropriately enjoys her position. When physicians discuss the nursing staff it would not be unusual for her name to be mentioned with respect and admiration. Their esteem for a good nurse is no less than their esteem for a good doctor.

The penalties for a game failure, on the other hand, can be severe. The physician who is an unskilled gamesman and fails to recognize the nurses' subtle recommendation messages is tolerated as a "clod." If, however, he interprets these messages as insolence and strongly indicates he does not wish to tolerate suggestions from nurses, he creates a rocky path for his travels.The old truism "If the nurse is your ally you've got it made, and if she has it in for you, be prepared for misery," takes on life-sized proportions. He receives three times as many phone calls after midnight than his colleagues. Nurses will not accept his telephone orders because "telephone orders are against the rules." Somehow, this rule gets suspended for the skilled players. Soon he becomes like Joe Bfstplk in the "Li'l Abner" comic strip. No matter where he goes, a black cloud constantly hovers over his head.

The unskilled gamesman nurse also pays heavily. The nurse who does not view her role as that of a consultant, and therefore does not attempt to communicate recommendations, is perceived as a dullard and is mercifully allowed to fade into the woodwork.

The nurse who does see herself as a consultant but refuses to follow the rules of the game in making her recommendations, has hell to pay. The outspoken nurse is labeled a "bitch" by the surgeon. The psychiatrist describes her as unconsciously suffering from penis envy and her behavior is the acting out of her hostility towards men. Loosely translated, the psychiatrist is saying she is a bitch. The employment of the unbright outspoken nurse is soon terminated. The outspoken bright nurse whose recommendations are worthwhile remains employed. She is, however, constantly reminded in a hundred ways that she is not loved.

GENESIS OF THE GAME

To understand how the game evolved, we must comprehend the nature of the doctors' and nurses' training which shaped the attitudes necessary for the game.

Medical Student Training

The medical student in his freshman year studies as if possessed. In the anatomy class he learns every groove and prominence on the bones of the skeleton as if life depended on it. As a matter of fact, he literally believes just that. He not infrequently says, "I've got to learn it exactly, a life may depend on me knowing that." A consequence of this attitude, which is carefully nurtured throughout medical school, is the development of a phobia: the overdetermined fear of making a mistake. The development of this fear is quite understandable. The burden the physician must carry is at times almost unbearable. He feels responsible in a very personal way for the lives of his patients. When a man dies leaving young children and a widow, the doctor carries some of her grief and despair inside himself; and when a child dies, some of him dies too. He sees himself as a warrior against death and disease. When he loses a battle, through no fault of his own, he nevertheless feels pangs of guilt, and he relentlessly searches himself to see if there might have been a way to alter the outcome. For the physician a mistake leading to a serious consequence is intolerable, and any mistake reminds him of his vulnerability. There is little wonder that he becomes phobic. The classical way in which phobias are managed is to avoid the source of the fear. Since it is impossible to avoid making some mistakes in an active practice of medicine, a substitute defensive maneuver is employed. The physician develops the belief that he is omnipotent and omniscient, and therefore incapable of making mistakes. This belief allows the phobic physician to actively engage in his practice rather than avoid it. The fear of committing an error in a critical field like medicine is unavoidable and appropriately realistic. The physician, however, must learn to live with the fear rather than handle it defensively through a posture of omnipotence. This defense markedly interferes with his interpersonal professional relationships.

Physicians, of course, deny feelings of omnipotence. The evidence, however, renders their denials to whispers in the wind. The slightest mistake inflicts a large narcissistic wound. Depending on his underlying personality structure the physician may obsess for days about it, quickly rationalize it away, or deny it. The guilt produced is usually exaggerated and the incident is handled defensively. The ways in which physicians enhance and support each other's defenses when an error is made could be the topic of another paper. The feelings of omnipotence become generalized to other areas of his life. A report of the Federal Aviation Agency (FAA), as quoted in *Time Magazine* (August 5, 1966), states that in 1964 and 1965 physicians had a fatal-accident rate four times as high as the average for all other private pilots. Major causes of the high death rate were risk-taking attitudes and judgments. Almost all of the accidents occurred on pleasure trips, and were therefore not necessary risks to get to a patient needing emergency care. The trouble, suggested an FAA official, is that too many doctors fly with "the feeling that they are omnipotent." Thus, the extremes to which the physician may go in preserving his self-concept of omnipotence may threaten his own life. This overdetermined preservation of omnipotence is indicative of its brittleness and its underlying foundation of fear of failure.

The physician finds himself trapped in a paradox. He fervently wants to give his patient the best possible medical care, and being open to the nurses' recommendations helps him accomplish this. On the other hand, accepting advice from nonphysicians is highly threatening to his omnipotence. The solution for the paradox is to receive sub rosa recommendations and make them appear to be initiated by himself. In short, he must learn to play the doctor–nurse game.

Some physicians never learn to play the game. Most learn in their internship, and a perceptive few learn during their clerkships in medical school. Medical students frequently complain that the nursing staff treats them as if they had just completed a junior Red Cross first-aid class instead of two years of intensive medical training. Interviewing nurses in a training hospital sheds considerable light on this phenomenon. In their words they said,

> A few students just seem to be with it, they are able to understand what you are trying to tell them and they are a pleasure to work with; most, however, pretend to know everything and refuse to listen to anything we have to say and I guess we do give them a rough time.

In essence, they are saying that those students who quickly learn the game are rewarded, and those that do not are punished.

Most physicians learn to play the game after they have weathered a few experiences like the one described below. On the first day of his internship, the physician and nurse were making rounds. They stopped at the bed of a 52-year-old woman who, after complimenting the young doctor on his appearance, complained to him of her problem with constipation. After several minutes of listening to her detailed description of peculiar diets, family home remedies, and special exercises that have helped her constipation in the past, the nurse politely interrupted the patient. She told her the doctor would take care of the problem and that he had to move on because there were other patients waiting to see him. The young doctor gave the nurse a stern look, turned toward the patient, and kindly told her he would order an enema for her that very afternoon. As they left the bedside, the nurse told him the patient has had a normal bowel movement every day for the past week and that in the 23 days the patient has been in the hospital she had never once passed up an opportunity to complain of her constipation. She quickly added that if the doctor wanted to order an enema, the patient would certainly receive one. After hearing this report the intern's mouth fell open and the wheels began turning in his head. He remembered the nurses comment to the patient that, "the doctor had to move on," and it occurred to him that perhaps she was really giving him a message. This experience and a few more like it, and the young doctor learns to listen for the subtle recommendations the nurses make.

Nursing Student Training

Unlike the medical student, who usually learns to play the game after he finishes medical school, the nursing student begins to learn it early in her training. Throughout her education she is trained to play the doctor–nurse game.

Student nurses are taught how to relate to physicians. They are told he has infinitely more knowledge than they, and thus he should be shown the utmost respect. In addition, it was not many years ago when nurses were instructed to stand whenever a physician entered a room. When he would come in for a conference the nurse was expected to offer him her chair, and when both entered a room the nurse would open the door for him and allow him to enter first. Although these practices are no longer rigidly adhered to, the premise upon which they were based is still promulgated. One nurse described that premise as, "He's God almighty and your job is to wait on him."

To inculcate subservience and inhibit deviancy, nursing schools, for the most part, are tightly run, disciplined institutions. Certainly there is great variation among nursing schools, and there is little question that the trend is toward giving students more autonomy. However, in too many schools this trend has not gone far enough, and the climate remains restrictive. The student's schedule is firmly controlled and there is very little free time. Classroom hours, study hours, meal time, and bedtime with lights out are rigidly enforced. In some schools meaningless chores are assigned, such as cleaning bed springs with cotton applicators. The relationship between student and instructor continues this military flavor. Often their relationship is more like that between recruit and drill sergeant than between student and teacher. Open dialogue is inhibited by attitudes of strict black and white, with few, if any, shades of gray. Straying from the rigidly outlined path is sure to result in disciplinary action.

The inevitable result of these practices is to instill in the student nurse a fear of independent action. This inhibition of independent action is most marked when relating to physicians. One of the students' greatest fears is making a blunder while assisting a physician and being publicly ridiculed by him. This is really more a reflection of the nature of their training than the prevalence of abusive physicians. The fear of being humiliated for a blunder while assisting in a procedure is generalized to the fear of humiliation for making any independent act in relating to a physician, especially the act of making a direct recommendation. Every nurse interviewed felt that making a suggestion to a physician was equivalent to insulting and belittling him. It was tantamount to questioning his medical knowledge and insinuating he did not know his business. In light of her image of the physician as an omniscient and punitive figure, the questioning of his knowledge would be unthinkable.

The student, however, is also given messages quite contrary to the ones described above. She is continually told that she is an invaluable aid to the physician in the treatment of the patient. She is told that she must help him in every way possible, and she is imbued with a strong sense of responsibility for the care of her patient. Thus she, like the physician, is caught in a paradox. The first set of messages implies that the physician is omniscient and that any recommendation she might make would be insulting to him and leave her open to ridicule. The second set of messages implies that she is an important asset to him, has much to contribute, and is duty-bound to make those contributions. Thus, when her good sense tells her a recommendation would be helpful to him she is not allowed to communicate it directly, nor is she allowed not to communicate it. The way out of the bind is to use the doctor–nurse game and communicate the recommendation without appearing to do so.

FORCES PRESERVING THE GAME

Upon observing the indirect interactional system which is the heart of the doctor–nurse game, one must ask the question, "Why does this inefficient mode of communication continue to exist?" The forces mitigating against change are powerful.

Rewards and Punishments

The doctor–nurse game has a powerful, innate self-perpetuating force—its system of rewards and punishments. One potent method of shaping behavior is to reward one set of behavioral patterns and to punish patterns which deviate from it. As described earlier, the rewards given for a well-played game and the punishments meted out to unskilled players are impressive. This system alone would be sufficient to keep the game flourishing. The game, however, has additional forces.

The Strength of the Set

It is well recognized that sets are hard to break. A powerful attitudinal set is the nurse's perception that making a suggestion to a physician is equivalent to insulting and belittling him. An example of where attempts are regularly made to break this set is seen on psychiatric treatment wards operating on a therapeutic community model. This model requires open and direct communication between members of the team. Psychiatrists working in these settings expend a great deal of energy in urging for and rewarding openness before direct patterns of communication become established. The rigidity of the resistance to break this set is impressive. If the physician himself is a prisoner of the set and therefore does not actively try to destroy it, change is near impossible.

The Need for Leadership

Lack of leadership and structure in any organization produces anxiety in its members. As the importance of the organization's mission increases, the demand by its members for leadership commensurately increases. In our culture human life is near the top of our hierarchy of values, and organizations which deal with human lives, such as law and medicine, are very rigidly structured. Certainly some of this is necessary for the systematic management of the task. The excessive degree of rigidity, however, is demanded by its members for their own psychic comfort rather than for its utility in efficiently carrying out its mission. The game lends support to this thesis. Indirect communication is an inefficient mode of transmitting information. However, it effectively supports and protects a rigid organizational structure with the physician in clear authority. Maintaining an omnipotent leader provides the other members with a great sense of security.

Sexual Roles

Another influence perpetuating the doctor–nurse game is the sexual identity of the players. Doctors are predominately men and nurses are almost exclusively women. There are elements of the game which reinforce the stereotyped roles of male dominance and female passivity. Some nursing instructors explicitly tell their students that their femininity is an important asset to be used when relating to physicians.

COMMENT

The doctor and nurse have a shared history and thus have been able to work out their game so that it operates more efficiently than one would expect in an indirect system. Major difficulty arises, however, when the physician works closely with other disciplines which are not normally considered part of the medical sphere. With expanding medical horizons encompassing cooperation with sociologists, engineers, anthropologists, computer analysts, etc., continued expectation of a doctor–nurselike interaction by the physician is disastrous. The sociologist, for example, is not willing to play that kind of game. When his direct communications are rebuffed the relationship breaks down.

The major disadvantage of a doctor–nurselike game is its inhibitory effect on open dialogue which is stifling and anti-intellectual. The game is basically a transactional neurosis, and both professions would enhance themselves by taking steps to change the attitudes which breed the game.

Structural Strain
in the Medical Marriage

Robert H. Coombs

Interpersonal strain is inherent in a medical marriage, regardless of the personalities involved. The overlapping statuses of physician and spouse, with their accompanying roles, are in a state of delicate balance and can easily be strained. When career and marriage become unbalanced, both domains suffer. But because the family is the most adaptive of all human institutions, problems at home typically occur first and are the most readily conspicuous.

The following discusses aspects of medical training and practice that most often exert stress on an intimate relationship. My information comes from lengthy tape-recorded interviews with academic physicians located at thirty different university teaching hospitals, mostly psychiatrists and obstetricians whose patient clientele includes physicians and their families. In what follows I use the masculine pronoun to refer to the doctor and the feminine to refer to his wife because, up to now, this has been by far the most typical configuration in the medical marriage. Nonetheless, the structural strains described here may be found in all medical marriages.

ABSENTEEISM DUE TO
PROFESSIONAL STATUS ANXIETIES

Since relationships of any type thrive upon rewarding interactions, minimizing shared experiences does little to promote feelings of

---

Some of the materials in this article have been adapted from my earlier writing on "The Medical Marriage" in Robert Coombs and C.E. Vincent (Eds.), *Psychosocial Aspects of Medical Training*. Springfield, Illinois: Charles C Thomas, 1971, pp. 133–166.

affection between family members. The potential for an "empty shell" marriage, one that is physically intact but psychologically impoverished, is great for the professional who becomes an absentee spouse.

There is strong potential for physicians to immerse themselves in their work to such an extent that they are rarely at home and when they are, to be absent in spirit. If not exhausted by the time they arrive home, they are likely to be preoccupied by their work—reading medical journals, mulling over the problems of the day, or contemplating those to be faced tomorrow.

Everyone knows, of course, that medical work can be demanding. In our society a very high priority is placed upon health, and doctors are expected, as "public servants," to drop everything else when called upon to heal. A good many of the physicians that I have interviewed, however, have pointed out that medical practice need not demand as much time as it typically does. To a larger extent than some will readily admit, medical practice tends to become, as one physician put it, a self-imposed life of exhaustion. That is, many of the demands are created internally by the physician. What accounts for these inner pressures?

Physicians, like others in our society, are accorded social honor on the basis of their performance in the work world; to be highly regarded requires a certain amount of occupational success. In addition, the recruitment system of medical education demands hard work. In order to earn the grades necessary for a place in medical school, an aspirant must be somewhat compulsive about studying.

Compulsive work habits become even more deeply ingrained in medical school. Surprisingly, freshmen medical students find that they have less status than they did in college. Having risen through successful competition to a position of prestige on the college campus, they become in medical school "the low person on the totem pole." This precipitous drop in status no doubt accounts for the frequent and sometimes bitter complaints from freshmen students about being "treated like children" or being viewed by the faculty as though they were "immature, unintellectual, and unmotivated." Hence, the need to prove themselves again.

Considerable anxiety is created by faculty members who grade by the traditional letter system, apparently assuming that medical students represent a normal distribution of intellectual abilities (which, obviously, they do not). Less than excellent grades is, for most medical students, a new experience. Small wonder that beginning students sometimes bury themselves in their work, even to the point, in some cases, of impairing physical and emotional health. Neither is it surprising that, when taking time off from their studies, they sometimes feel guilty or are haunted by the image of their classmates "booking it" while they fall behind.

The drive to be successful, of course, is not unique to those who choose medicine as their career. Few other careers, however, seem to create as much status anxiety. The see-saw course of medical training recurrently strips young people of much of their hard-earned status and starts them at the bottom again. Students or resident physicians barely achieve one height, one peak in their careers, before they have to begin again as fledglings and prove themselves anew. In few occupations does a person intermittently occupy the position of neophyte over such a long period. Even after one's residency is completed, there are board examinations to pass, a practice to be built, and a reputation to be established.

To an outsider, it would seem that young people "arrive" when they graduate from medical school and become physicians. Within medical circles, however, this is just the beginning. The young doctors, of course, gain satisfaction from family, friends, and others in the community who acknowledge their hard-earned medical degrees, but they look to other physicians for their concept of self-worth as physicians. They have become a reference group—one which evaluates by standards of excellence. There is little opportunity to rest on one's laurels, because there are always new emergencies to cope with, new knowledge to acquire, and new techniques to master. It is small wonder that conscientious physicians are described as "perpetual students." Neither is it surprising that many are willing to sacrifice personal pleasures and to neglect family affairs in the interest of the "sacred doctor-patient relationship"; for this dedication, by according them prestige among their colleagues, gives them self-esteem.

STATUS OF DOCTOR'S SPOUSE
AS COMPARED WITH OTHERS

When the medical student marries, both bride and groom are usually on about the same intellectual and social level. But while the student is experiencing tremendous personal and intellectual growth through contact with stimulating people and an exposure to a variety of complicated things, the spouse may remain at about the same level, especially if in putting the student-mate through school she is tied down to an uncreative job, or is largely confined to the home if children are involved. Although the spouse may wish to expand in a sphere of activity and knowledge, children and a lack of funds may prohibit a very wide range of personal experiences.

One physician described the situation this way: "He married her when they were both frumps. But he went up and she stayed a frump." Another made a similar observation: "These two caterpillars married when they were in college and one of them turned into a butterfly but the other one remained a caterpillar. You've got to bring the other caterpillar along. It's only fair."

In medical practice, the doctor meets many people of the opposite sex who are educated and sophisticated and have taken pains before leaving home to make themselves attractive and to display their best behavior. In returning home, however, the physician often finds a harried spouse whose faults and limitations are well known and who shows the strain of the work day, and sometimes of raising small children. Quite naturally a comparison may be made of the spouse, at her worst, with others of the same sex who have been seen at their best. Hence, as one physician explained, "When physicians go into practice they are drawn even further away from the now 'dowdy' spouse by the more sophisticated associates they interact with. These others appear more attractive and more socially acceptable than the 'little mouse of a spouse' who has stuck in there all those years." Consequently, the physican may feel trapped in a boring marriage and have the desire to escape.

STATUS DEPRIVATION
OF THE DOCTOR AT HOME

It is no secret that doctors enjoy very high status and are accorded admiration and respect, not only by their patients in medical contexts, but by those in other settings as well. In few other professions is a person's occupational status generalized to such an extent. Wherever physicians go, they are greeted as "Doc" and are viewed, it seems, as having knowledge and expertise on nearly every topic. A glimpse of oneself in such a favorable "looking glass" no doubt does marvelous things for one's self-image, and it is easy to understand how a physician can "get drunk on his own juices" and come to expect deference from others.

But, alas, the one place where a doctor is least likely to be treated as "doctor" is at home. Being accustomed to a privileged status in society, the physician may find it degrading to come home and be asked to take out the garbage or to perform other menial tasks which, in medical contexts, are regarded as "scut work." Because of long intimate association, the physician is not likely to be perceived by the spouse as Dr. Butterfly, but instead as simply Joe or Mary Caterpillar. That is, the spouse responds to the doctor as a total person rather than as a professional per se.

The doctor may be deprived of status not only by having to drop the Dr. Butterfly role when returning home, but also by having a "frumpish" spouse waiting as a reminder of the "Doc's" own frumpish, caterpillar origins. This status deprivation may be further exaggerated if, out of resentment for neglect of family matters, the spouse rallies the children against the doctor-parent. Such a situation increases the likelihood of the physician becoming resentful and withdrawing even further from family activities. Most physicians find it is more rewarding to stay at work receiving mass adoration—the deference of patients and others—than to fight it out with the unappreciative little group of people at home.

RESISTANCE IN RECOGNIZING AND SEEKING HELP FOR FAMILY PROBLEMS

Many patients attribute almost superhuman knowledge and abilities to their doctor. This supernatural aura is probably related to the fact that patients must develop a kind of blind faith in their physician. When allowing another person to hold your life in the balance while surgery is taking place, for example, or to influence your health in any way, the last thing you want to do is to doubt the competence of that person. Under such conditions, it is psychologically natural to *want* to believe in the doctor's infallibility.

In an attempt to maintain an image of high competence and certitude, a physician may tend to avoid an objective recognition of personal failings. One psychiatrist called this "the doctor's blind spot." "Because they're experts in their field, they tend to think they can do no wrong. They feel some sort of immunity, not realizing that they too can rationalize."

It is painful and embarrassing for all human beings to acknowledge personal failure, and the pain is probably exaggerated for those who are cast in the role of possessing more than human qualities. Can a healer who is not whole be trusted any more than a driver-education teacher whose automobile has dented fenders, or a finance advisor who is not prosperous? Although it is unreasonable to assume that doctors, or anybody else, should be exempt from having human qualities, there is pressure, as a psychiatrist put it, "to feel that you must be a paragon of mental health."

It is natural for all human beings to develop ego defenses for personal failures. A ready defense for doctors is to accept and internalize patients' attitudes toward them, so that they become convinced of their own infallibility. Personal and family problems can then be explained away as somebody else's fault. It is interesting to note that the public tends to support doctors in this defense. It never occurs to most people that the doctor might be partly responsible for the spouse's emotional problems. Instead, the reaction usually seems to be, "The poor doctor still carries on in helping others in spite of personal burdens."

When marital conflicts arise, a physician may choose to play the same role with the spouse as is done with patients—namely, maintaining a nonemotional, directive manner and simply not tolerating any conflict. In other words, the physician can withdraw emotionally, and perhaps physically as well. In maintaining emotional equilibrium with patients, it is impossible to take on the emotional burden of each one. In this way the clinician shields inner feelings from others' problems. This "detached concern" may serve doctors well in their clinical roles, but may work against them in marriage.

If a physician is willing to assume some responsibility for an unhealthy marriage, there may be reservations about sharing this problem with medical colleagues or with other helping professionals, since they are likely to be acquaintances. Because there is a good deal of defensive competitive pride between professionals, it requires considerable humility and courage for a physician to seek assistance. Many doctors, therefore, rather than attempting to reverse the unhealthy trend of their marriages through counseling, find it easier to ignore or rationalize the problem as someone else's problem, and become more deeply immersed in medical practice.

PRIORITY OF MEDICAL NEEDS
OVER FAMILY NEEDS

In our society families are expected to adapt to the changing demands of career. Because of the very high value placed upon health, the families of physicians are expected to be especially adaptable. In fact, medical practice provides a ready escape from almost any situation. An ordinary person would be considered rude when leaving a banquet in the middle of the dessert course or a theater party during Act II. In the case of a physician, however, others assume the departure is for a hospital emergency. Trying to capitalize on such tolerance, others have masqueraded as physicians in order to avoid speeding tickets.

Physicians who consistently spend long hours at their work are generally applauded by the public, for it is assumed that they are sacrificing themselves for the benefit of humanity. Those more familiar with the hospital setting, however, may note that some doctors, rather than going home, spend much of their time chatting, drinking coffee, or playing ping-pong in the doctors' lounge. As one indicated, "Some doctors just never go home; you become aware that they are trying to avoid the evening or weekend at home." Other physicians who show an abnormal devotion to work are trying to get ahead professionally. An obstetrician explained:

> The doctor can get into a situation where more and more people want the services and refusal becomes impossible. However, I believe that the doctor's own desire to do this, at least subconsciously, accounts for a large part of this. I realize that this is not the most popular viewpoint, but medical practice is like business or academic work: to get to the top takes so much energy that one has to sacrifice everything else. Now, the difference in medicine is that the doctor has a better excuse for putting spouse and family second if desired.

When at home, a physician may continue to use the medical role for escaping unpleasant aspects of family interaction. From personal experience, a divorced physician confided that medicine is sometimes used as an excuse for not engaging in marital sexual relations. "How do you expect me to have sex with you when I've got to worry about So-and-So who's dying?" Physicians involved in extramarital affairs have an advantageous situation, for they can come and go as they wish and receive phone calls at any hour of the night or day, and still be viewed as noble. Among all the other professions, only clergymen seem to have such a ready-made excuse for their behavior. Who can find fault with those who are involved in humane services, whether "engaged in the Lord's work" or in delivering babies, reducing pain, and in other ways improving the human condition?

CONCLUSION

No evidence exists that physicians have less stable marriages than other couples. In fact, what little data there are available suggest just the opposite. But the potential for a psychologically impoverished relationship is great when physicians devote themselves fully to career and are unaware of the built-in strain that exists between the overlapping roles of physician and spouse-parent. Sensitive awareness and thoughtful effort are required if one is to maintain a viable and healthy balance between the two.

A Physician's Prologue to Retirement

William J. Perry

Physicians approaching retirement or semiretirement will eventually face to some degree an emotional response to this change, including equating the loss of practice with the loss of status. The response will vary with the intensity of the person's previous dedication to medicine, current mental and physical status, and misgivings regarding both the good and bad in his or her practice years. Some will weather this transposition without overt emotional decay. For me, the hiatus between the two phases of my life seemed interminable, but once the decision was made, I knew it was best not to look back.

"There is no heavier burden than a great opportunity." This roadside sign, without advertising, stood majestically atop a hillside on a secure pedestal, as if to amplify its meaning and lend credence to its text. The words haunted me during my emotional travel north up the interstate to investigate a position removed from the pressures of solo practice. The journey was my first step in preparing for semiretirement. I was looking forward to shorter and less complicated work days, vacations that could be enjoyed without mentally calculating the monetary loss caused by being away from the office, and the freedom my wife and I would mutually enjoy with this new endeavor. The temptation to turn south, however, back toward home was nearly overwhelming, for that sunken feeling of loneliness for what I was leaving behind could not be relieved even by the thought and expectation of a "great opportunity."

The scale between burden and great opportunity was not balanced at this stage of the venture. The anonymous quotation from the sign has or will have great meaning to those approaching voluntary retirement in comfort or involuntary retirement due to unfortunate circumstances. Retirement is the beginning of a great burden—psychologically, financially, and physically. I know I can't make up to myself, and especially not to my family, the many impositions of the past 30 years. The nature of medical practice instills within physicians a strong inclination to continue to practice despite, and at times at the expense of, family need. I could not remedy that acid feeling as I drove along.

Amid the seeming confusion of our medical world, physicians are so nicely adjusted to a system—and systems to one another and to a whole—that by stepping aside to a new adventure, they expose themselves to the fearful risk of losing their identity and place forever. The risk may contribute to the agonizing preadjustment of retirement. I have a feeling that no one will be immune to this agony as time goes by.

Most of us do some financial planning, although never enough. It seemed that no matter how many hours I worked per week, my expected contribution to retirement never met the four- or five-digit figure suggested by financial planners. If current retirees find their financial assets inadequate, it's probably due in part to the drastic economic upheaval that they could not anticipate and plan for. Planning needs to be more aggressive for today's physician.

When "leaving practice" is first announced at staff meetings, you are greeted with multiple expressions of "it takes a lot of guts to do that today" or "I wish I could land a job like that" or "you deserve a break." I'm not sure what the real feelings are behind these different comments. Happy to expect overflow patients? Happy to see a less stringent review coordinator for medical records? Or are they feelings of sympathy for a past illness that may have a prospective poor prognosis? In any case, they are offered with mixed emotions and, under the circumstances, taken from those few friends that come by years of tolerance.

From that day on, while completing unfinished business around town, you feel like an extra thumb in a five-finger glove. You feel detached from the bond and excitement of the patient–physician–hospital relationship. You may be missed by the hospital and nursing staff on a scale commensurate with your importance to local medicine and colleagues. Now is the day of judgment! For me, it was difficult. I enjoyed my association with the nursing personnel, typist, admitting clerk, medical records team, cooks, and bookkeepers. It was a refreshing routine for me to pickup my own X-ray films and duplicate progress notes in morning rounds. These tasks brought bits of conversation that carried everyone's friendliness to the next day.

Hospital gossip added to the spice of friendship. A friendly reminder about my scribbled orders and somewhat illegible progress notes, the tagging of a chart that shows overutilization by one day, and the echoes of medical staff gripes that change little over the years will not be a part of a new career.

Our move to a smaller house means elimination of prized items that can't be used due to limited space. The ol' band saw, drill press, and radial arm saw are too big to fit comfortably in the new home. There are drawers filled with tacks, glass knobs, sawdust, and one-of-a-kind items to be used "later." Much of this hadn't been missed for years, but the memories of how each was collected bring fleeting escape to yesterday. The workshop becomes quieter and colder. Everything about me demonstrates a careless desolation.

Several times my wife emerges and breaks the silence with a photo or two of temporarily forgotten moments of fun, or she holds up some nondescript item to see if it is recognizable enough to save. Most were found in boxes of "junk" that had not seen a cleaning hand for years. What to get rid of? What to save? Will the children want anything? We had already saved the youngsters' crib that had lost its bearings, then the springs, and finally the more important guardrails. Although it couldn't possibly be salvaged, we add it to the packing list.

I was not prepared for these decisions. It was a burden I couldn't accept, but my wife had made up her mind to be content in our new venture—masking hidden feelings, I'm sure—and worked away like a galley slave. No tribute is great enough for her encouragement to me and her facing the closing ordeal. Even then I had not come to terms with my own ambivalence (and related guilt) about not continuing to practice until I was more feeble than a majority of my patients.

There were lonely thoughts and reflections—somehow coming too late—on the ups and downs of private practice and the sacrifices made by our family. I recalled the number of times an anxious face wanted to go camping, take a short vacation, or go to a movie. As I drive north with the percussion sounds of passing fence posts and the whine of tires on asphalt, the feeble reply keeps mentally recurring: "I can't take the time this week. We'll have to do it later." Time lost is never found again. There is no backtracking. All the proverbs about time wasted and things to be done yesterday can't be fulfilled today. However, I do look forward to tomorrow and hope to share experiences with a now-grown family and older parent to partially make up for my inequities in days past as a busy physician.

Dag Hammarskjöld aptly put these feelings in perspective, providing an appropriate aphorism for us all: "We carry our nemesis within us. Yesterday's self-admiration is the legitimate father of today's feeling of guilt."

RECOMMENDED READING

Medical Practice

Angell, Marcia, 1983, "Women in Medicine: Beyond Prejudice," *The New England Journal of Medicine*, Vol. 304, No. 19, pp. 1161–1162.

Berman, Ellen M., 1980, *Adult Development and the Physician's Marriage*, (formerly: "The Physician's Marriage, Joys and Sorrows, Part 2: Life Transition Points," *Facets*, Winter, 1979), Marriage Council of Philadelphia, Inc.

Burnam, John F., 1984, "The Unfortunate Case of Dr. Z: How to Succeed in Medical Practice in 1984," *The New England Journal of Medicine*, Vol. 310, No. 11, pp. 729–730.

Carey, Susan, 1984, "Foreign Doctors Fill a Medical-Care Gap in Backwater Towns," *The Wall Street Journal*, May 23, 1984.

Freedman, Steve A., "Megacorporate Health Care: A Choice for the Future," *New England Journal of Medicine*, Vol. 312, No. 9, pp. 579–582.

Groves, James E., 1978, "Taking Care of the Hateful Patient," *The New England Journal of Medicine*.

Guze, Samuel B., 1979, "Can the Practice of Medicine Be Fun For a Lifetime?" *Journal of the American Medical Association*, Vol. 241, No. 19, pp. 2021–2023.

LaSalle, Gar., 1982, "Emergency Medicine: Notes on an Undeciphered Diary," *Cornell University Medical College Alumni Quarterly*, Vol. 44, No. 2, pp. 14–17.

McCue, Jack D., 1982, "The Effects of Stress on Physicians and Their

Medical Practice," *The New England Journal of Medicine*, Vol. 306, No. 8, pp. 458–463.

McCue, Jack D., 1982, *Private Practice: Surviving the First Year*, Heath and Company, Lexington, Mass., 285 pages.

Nadelson, Theodore, and Eisenberg, Leon, 1977, "The Successful Professional Woman: On Being Married to One," *The American Journal of Psychiatry*, Vol. 134, No. 10, pp. 1071–1076.

Osborne, David, 1984, "My Wife the Doctor," *Mother Jones*, January Issue, pp. 21–25, 42–45.

Decline and Retirement

Howard, Robert B., 1983, "Physicians as Patients: The Lessons of Experience," *Postgraduate Medicine*, Vol. 74, No. 2, pp. 15–19.

Lunsford, Thomas E., 1981, "Problems of the Aging Physician: A Report of the Commission on Physician Impairment," *The Journal of the Indiana State Medical Association*, Vol. 74, No. 12, pp. 778–779.

Mullan, Fitzhugh, 1975, "A Diagnosis: A Doctor Turned Patient Measures Medicine's Vital Signs," *Vital Signs*, reprinted in *The New Physician*, No. 3, 1983.

Rabin, David, and Roni, Pauline L., 1982, "Compounding the Ordeal of ALS: Isolation from My Fellow Physician," *Journal of Medicine*, Vol. 307, No. 8, pp. 506–509.

Sargent, Douglas A., 1982, "Vignette: Post-Thoracotomy Cryoangalgesia: A Physician's Personal Experience," *Psychiatric Annals*, Vol. 12, No. 71, pp. 726–727.

Thomas, Lewis, 1983, "Diagnosing the Doctor: A Physician Turned Patient Gets Some Illuminating Lessons in Hospital Procedure and Anatomy (his own)," *Readers Digest*, November 1983, pp. 185–188 (condensed from *The Youngest Science: Notes of a Medicine-Watcher*, Viking Press, New York, pp. 185–188).

Wilbourn, Asa J., 1972, "A Report on the Infection in My Head," *Hospital Physician*, March Issue, pp. 38–40, 63–64.

II

DEVELOPMENTAL OUTCOMES

4

Impaired Physicians: Wasted Potential

It is ironic that anybody trained to be a health professional should lose his or her own health in the process. Yet this is what happens to some physicians. Depression, substance abuse, and even suicide are not beyond the realm of potential experience. Physicians are human too.

It is well documented that many members of the medical profession suffer from emotional distress that affects not only their work but other areas of their lives as well. Gross impairment is usually preceded by depleted energy, job dissatisfaction, and professional incompetence. As clinical standards fall and quality of work is compromised, negative attitudes develop toward patients, colleagues, and associates—and finally toward self. Strained relationships develop at home as well as at work.

Emotional impairment in the medical profession first became an issue of widespread concern in 1972 when the American Medical Association's Council on Mental Health issued its landmark statement on "the sick physician." Since then, there has been a proliferation of programs throughout the country to deal with impaired physicians. Sponsored by local medical societies and hospitals, these programs have been designed to detect, confront, and provide rehabilitation services. In nearly every state, medical societies now have impaired physician committees and, since 1975, the AMA has sponsored a bi-annual national conference on the topic of impairment and has circulated throughout the country an AMA Impaired Physician Newsletter.

In an inaugural address, a recent AMA president urged physicians to take action on behalf of their troubled colleagues. "If a physician knows a colleague who becomes impaired . . .," he said, "that physican should be willing to personally express concern and to encourage the impaired physician to seek help. . . . If the persuasion needs to be a bit more pointed, each physician should recognize that this, too, involves his or her individual responsibility to the profession, as well as to the errant colleague."

Stress intrinsic to the physician's work has typically been held accountable for emotional impairment. One author has catalogued these stressors as day-to-day encounters with patient suffering, fear, sexuality, and death; pervasive uncertainty in dealing with medical problems and interpersonal difficulties created by such problems.

We do not deny, of course, the well-established link between stress and emotional or physical disorders. Nor do we discount the fact that medical trainees/physicians experience considerable stress, some of which may be dysfunctional to their role performance. But, to attribute physician impairment to stress seems oversimplified. Such reasoning fails to recognize that some stressors—those that are role-relevant—are precursors to professional and personal development and, if handled successfully, can foster feelings of progress and fulfillment rather than the opposite. Such a view also ignores the fact that prospective physicians, having had glimpses of medical drama at medical centers through personal contact as well as the mass media, are attracted to the physician's career precisely for these reasons—they want a rewarding career that promises stimulating challenges and exhilarating experiences, those deemed significant and important by society.

Emotional problems among physicians and other professionals who have selected "open-ended careers" (i.e., those with relatively great freedom to decide the schedule of their work hours) result, in our view, not from too much stress, but from dysfunctional methods of coping. In the pursuit of excellence, in constantly trying to prove one's competence by impressing a critical audience (primarily other physicians), the doctor's lifestyle can easily become unbalanced, skewed in the direction of career attainment. Such individuals, chronically overworked and preoccupied with work-related matters, can become physically and emotionally exhausted, with anxiety, irritability, and depression as predictable manifestations. This condition is exacerbated when, in order to appear competent and strong, they also chronically suppress personal feelings of anxiety, doubt, and inadequacy, emotions that cry for expression. Such physicians become excellent candidates for emotional impairment.

Unrealistic expectations, overwork, and emotional isolation seem to be at the core of physician impairment.

Entering medical students are often surprised and disillusioned by what they find at medical school—status deprivation, relatively poor quality teaching, and the seemingly clinical irrelevance of materials they are required to learn. But there is no gap between their expectations and the reality that hard work is required in order to master the materials (Coombs and Boyle, 1971). They fully expect and are already "programmed" by their pre-med training to put in long hours.

The recruitment process favors those who are willing to work hard, to sacrifice personal pleasures in order to obtain the credentials necessary for admission manifested by high scholastic grades and MCAT scores. Such individuals are extraordinarily motivated for career success. Rather than floundering in search of a meaningful career like so many of their youthful peers, most medical students decide to be physicians at an early age. Even before entering college, three out of five in one longitudinal study population (Coombs, 1978) had clear vision of a medical career; 21 percent could not ever recall a time that they had not wanted to be a physician. Moreover, when asked what career they would have selected had medical school been inaccessible, more than three-fourths (76 percent) could not think of an alternative career.

Excessive work results not only from faculty demands, but from their own competitiveness, thoroughness, and idealism. Trainees worry that if the materials are not mastered, later on someone might die because of their ignorance. Consequently, recreational and social life, so essential for mental health, often take the form of "binges." At all stages of training—during medical school, internship, and residency—trainees report that they not only work hard, they also "play hard." Work schedules of as many as 120 hours per week are reported by some clinicians, leaving seven hours a day for all other activities, including sleep. Sleep deprivation has been demonstrated to affect psychological well-being. Small wonder that nonphysician observers, like the author of one of our selections, have asked whether such training is "preparation or hazing."

The problems created by overwork are exacerbated by a conduct norm that equates professionalism with emotional inexpressiveness. In medical settings, good clinicians are well in control of their emotions at all times. When judged by this norm, each trainee, secretly feeling anxiously overwhelmed, develops a profound sense of personal inadequacy. Hundreds of hours of personal interviews with medical trainees have made clear these anxieties and self-doubts. Although almost everyone feels this way, each trainee thinks that he or she is the only one so afflicted. So, by projecting a calm exterior like their mentors, they become emotionally isolated.

Despite this ubiquitous problem, relatively little is done to encourage appropriate emotional expressiveness. Instead, neophyte clinicians are expected to remain analytical and emotionally aloof. In their male-dominated milieu, such composure—machismo—is highly valued. To openly express personal feelings among scientifically oriented associates is to risk the appearance of being "soft" or "weak," in short, "nonprofessional."

This is readily apparent in anatomy and autopsy rooms where human bodies are dissected with apparent equanimity. As an adaptive technique, trainees learn to suppress or intellectualize their feelings. The challenge for the neophyte clinician is to privately maintain personal sensitivity while publicly carving on a human body.

As Finkelstein's article has demonstrated, rather than recognizing the urgent need for emotional exploration and expression, little is done to provide structural opportunities. As such, this developmental task is essentially ignored, avoided, or suppressed. Coupled with self-doubt, constantly demanding work, and chronic fatigue, emotional impairment is enhanced.

These points are exemplified by a female resident who shares her deepest feelings.

> The major problem that I have is lack of time and energy. I can remember feeling fatigued when I was a medical student, but it wasn't the extreme fatigue that I feel now.
>
> I was brought up on the idea that all women should get married, have their kiddies, settle down into a snug little home. When you're exhausted, and don't even have control over that aspect of life, sometimes you get to feeling a little suicidal. I know other women physicians who have confided about extreme depression, just almost unable to function at all. This is because we feel that we don't have anyone who cares, no family that's able to provide support. It gets really depressing when you feel exhausted and don't have anyone close to share your feelings with. I think that most of the suicides that occur among physicians come at a time in life when they had no emotional support, too much stress, and too few close associates to pull them through.
>
> I had a close personal friend who, I learned to my horror, was abusing drugs, and I just couldn't understand how anyone could do that. But after being an intern I learned. After I was three or four months into my internship I started thinking, "I've got to

somehow stop this misery and horror. I just can't stand it any longer. What can I do?" I looked around and noticed that there were lots of drugs available. Then I caught myself. How could I have even thought of that? I resisted, probably because I can't stand being injected with needles. But now I understand how people get into that trap. It's a very bad trap. You really get into danger when you're sleep deprived and keep your feelings inside. When you live with a lot of stresses and pressures it's important to relieve the tension by talking with someone. I usually keep my mouth shut among acquaintances that I don't know all that well. But I can talk it out with good friends. I'll come up and say, "blah, blah, blah," and they'll reply, "Yeah, I know. It's a drag." And that relieves some tension. If you keep things locked up inside, you find yourself either starting to scream at people, like I do, or else get very depressed and become suicidal, the way other people do. It's a very dangerous situation.

We have chosen John Rhoads' article as the first selection because, as the title indicates, it deals with "overwork," a common problem among physicians and others who have open-ended careers with no set hours. Overwork is defined by Rhoads as "working beyond one's endurance and capacities." Some individuals, he notes, lack an inner governor to regulate a healthy balance between work, rest, and recreation. "Cursed with a compulsive need to work," he says, "they deny the existence of fatigue and push themselves beyond reason." Unable to concentrate, distractible, and drowsy, they drive themselves to complete the task in time, often lengthening their workday to compensate for their lessened ability to produce efficiently. Recuperative power is diminished when, in order to meet work demands, exercise and recreation are eliminated. Clusters of symptoms may then develop—fatigue, irritability, sleep disturbances, memory lapse, depression, and various physical ailments. Rhoads points out that overwork among physicians is exacerbated by fear of failure and the need to be loved by everyone.

Personal problems inevitably become worse when, in order to keep going, physicians medicate themselves or turn to alcoholic beverages for relief. To illustrate this gradual deterioration, we have selected a moving personal account of a "recovering addict" whose problems began in his residency, when he sought "chemical pep" to get him through the long hours and "brutal pace." "I'm a Doctor—and a Drug Addict" describes one physician's increasing use of chemicals and the personal/professional decline that ensued. Fortunately, this anonymous physician eventually found his way to a drug rehabilitation program especially designed for physicians, and currently he assists others with problems of chemical dependency. Now, he points out, "When I suffer from fatigue, I'll be tempted by my prescription pad. But I won't be alone anymore. A network of recovering addictionologists, therapists and recovering addicts will be ready to help me out. All I have to do is ask."

Unfortunately, happy endings don't always occur when physicans abuse themselves. Rather than seeking and finding competent professional help, some become more and more exhausted, depressed, and isolated. The tragic story of one talented young physician who ended her life during her internship is told in the next selection by her bereaved mother. In hopes of helping others avoid the degeneration processes of medical training, Erika Rosemark courageously shares an intimate account of her daughter's overwhelming experiences as an intern. After offering a list of excellent suggestions for monitoring the well-being of physican trainees, she asks, "How can physicans whose own health and happiness is being ignored, adequately treat their patients with compassion and concern?"

"Why does the medical profession not do a better job of preventing suicide among its members than it does?" is a related question, one asked by Douglas A. Sargent and his colleague in their article, "Preventing Physician Suicide: The Role of Family, Colleagues, and Organized Medicine." In this article the authors point out the psychological barriers to suicide prevention. Physicians in presuicidal states, they note, often refuse to seek help because of their own delusions of infallibility, a failure that is reinforced by worshipful attitudes by family and patients. For the same reasons, physician colleagues tend to deny "weakness" or react with annoyance when confronted, masking an accurate self-assessment of suicidal feelings. By the time the depressed physican reaches treatment, if at all, family members, friends, and colleagues may have been alienated and personal funds exhausted. Submitting to a colleague or accepting "professional courtesy" further challenges physician self-esteem.

The final article, "When Doctors Fail to Care for Themselves," by George Vaillant, is adapted from a lecture given to medical students at Harvard Medical School. We included it here because it discusses the coping strategies typically utilized by physicians under stress, unconscious adaptive styles sometimes referred to as "ego mechanisms of defense." The author highlights interesting examples of physician altruism, reaction formation, passive-aggression, and dissociation (neurotic denial) and provides important suggestions for their appropriate utilization.

Vaillant urges students to develop wisdom, to be rational in the face of irrational feelings and behavior. "In order to deal with normal slings and arrows," he states, "doctors tend to use certain defense mechanisms more than others, and understanding them can help you pay attention to getting care for yourself in order to care for others." "Physican," he urges, "cherish thyself."

REFERENCES

Coombs, R. H., 1978, "Mastering Medicine: Professional Socialization in Medical School," Free Press/Macmillan, New York.

Coombs, R. H., and Boyle, B. P., 1971, "The Transition to Medical School: Expectations versus Realities," *Psychosocial Aspects of Medical Training*, Charles C Thomas, Springfield, Illinois, pp. 91–109.

Overwork

John M. Rhoads

To the internist or family physician, fatigue is probably the most commonly voiced complaint. It is often attributed to overwork, but seldom is this a correct diagnosis. In fact, it is almost axiomatic that if a patient complains of being overworked, he is not. Such a complaint was likely to be true in the early days of the Industrial Revolution, when work weeks ranged from 60 to 80 hours, and the seven-day week was the rule. At present, when the 40-hour week is standard, and where a 26-hour week is standard for one craft union in the nation's largest city, it may be surprising that anyone is overworked.

However, there are special groups of individuals who are susceptible to overwork. These people continue in the mode of the last century, when the working man labored from sunrise to sunset and beyond. No employer would be allowed to work his employees to such an excess. The exceptions are self employers who occupy open-ended positions. This group includes business executives, lawyers, doctors, accountants, clergymen, and occasionally even housewives.

Members of this group consult a physician, not with a complaint of overwork, but rather with the complaint that they are unable to work as long and as well as they feel they should. This is usually an incidental complaint, the chief complaint being one of a variety of physical symptoms. Symptoms may be quite variable, depending on the state or degree of exhaustion, the symbolic importance of particular symptoms, and chance. They commonly include fatigue, irritability, sleep disturbances, difficulty concentrating, memory lapses, confusional episodes, depression, gastrointestinal malfunctions, cardiovascular disturbances, or neuromuscular complaints.

Most persons in executive positions or professions or who are self-employed are able to pace themselves by balancing their drive, energy, and recuperative capacity against the realistic demands of the job and the goals they require of themselves. While occasionally they must overextend themselves, they learn to compensate to maintain the expenditure-recuperation equilibrium.

Some persons seem to lack an inner monitoring device for regulating the work-rest-recreation balance. Cursed with a compulsive need to work, they deny the existence of fatigue and push themselves beyond reason. They attempt to cope with diminished ability to concentrate, ease of distractibility, and drowsiness (early signs of fatigue) by forcing themselves to stay at the appointed task. In fact, they usually lengthen the workday to compensate for their lessened ability to produce efficiently. This self-prescription only accentuates the problem, since not only do they become more tired, but they usually will eliminate exercise or recreation time, further diminishing their recuperative capacity. Similarly, necessary extensions of recuperation time because of aging are ignored, so that one often finds such persons in their 60s attempting to maintain their schedule of 40 years ago.

From these early symptoms, the syndrome progresses to memory lapses, confusion, and depression, and may mimic anxiety reactions, myocardial infarctions, or even organic brain syndromes. Their family may have cautioned them, though in many instances, they seem to have chosen cooperative spouses who willingly tolerate their neglect of family life. As children do not have this option, they tend to suffer more from the problem of the parent. In some instances, the families have urged the correct treatment on the patient, only to find that the patient angrily rejects the proffered help, since the cure makes him feel all the more guilty.

The following cases are examples of overwork occurring in a variety of occupations and in different types of persons.

REPORT OF CASES

* * *

Case 3

A 52-year-old physician, a general practitioner in a small town, was referred by his wife, who was fearful he might commit suicide. His principal complaints were depression, difficulty concentrating, episodes of confusion and poor memory, tension and anxiety of four to five months' duration, chronic fatigue, unhappiness, inability to enjoy life, and a 3-kg weight loss in the past several months. He was unable to date the onset of his illness but knew that it had been building up for at least six months. He noted that he had doubled his usual consumption of cigarettes, found that he was waking up too early in the morning, and would lie in bed fretting about financial problems, aging, Medicare, the government, assorted patients, and the state of his health. He feared that he would require electroconvulsive therapy or would have to retire. Aproximately one year previously, he had had a similar episode but felt better after his wife convinced him to take her on a four-day vacation. He insisted that he was unable to take any time off, since he was behind in his work, was building a new house, and needed to stay at work to be able to pay for it. He insisted that he had many very sick patients who required his presence. He had attempted self-medication with oxazepam, which further decreased his ability to think clearly. He had not taken a vacation for years, except as previously noted. He estimated that his practice took about 60 hours a week, not counting emergencies and night calls. In addition, he was active in civic affairs, so that he was out nearly every night in the week. He had dropped all exercise and recreation from his schedule. He was persuaded to take a two-week vacation with his family and returned much improved. He resumed his practice but dropped several of his extra jobs and substituted an active recreational program.

Three years later, he was seen again because of severe depression. This time, the history disclosed a period preceding the depression of overwork, unsound financial ventures, excessive energy and euphoria. He was treated successfully for the depression with amitriptyline hydrochloride, 150 mg daily, and then received maintenance doses of lithium carbonate. He has been well for four years. In this case, a diagnosis of manic-depressive illness was made, one manifestation of the illness being the overwork syndrome.

Case 4

A 54-year-old physician, a general practitioner in a small agricultural town, complained of depression, which he noted had been building for several years. His work schedule typically consisted of seven days a week with no time off, and his last vacation was seven years ago. He had lost interest in work, lacked his usual good humor, was worried, had midnight wakening with inability to go back to sleep, a weight loss of 11 kg, low energy, loss of libido, and constipation.

Of crucial importance was the fact that the patient was the only black physician in the area. The local physicians, of whom there were a dozen or so, proposed to him a division of the patient population of the county, namely that they would take care of the white patients, and he the black. However, he would rotate with them on emergency calls at the local hospital. This left him with the entire black population (approximately 10,000 patients), a regular rotation on the emergency call schedule, and no one to take backup calls from his patients. The result was that he was working long hours, with a low income since most of his patients were rural, poor, and not covered by insurance. His dedication to his patients accounted in large measure for his overwork and for recurring financial problems. Fortunately, local attitudes had improved since the original arrangement, and he was able to work out a more equitable apportionment of the work load.

ATTITUDES TOWARD WORK

It may be helpful at this point to review attitudes toward work expressed by a variety of persons. These give general agreement on the value of work, modest agreement as to its virtue, and little as to how much work is enough.

Freud[1] saw work as a basis for attaching the individual firmly to reality, "work ... gives him a secure place in a portion of reality in the human community." He added not only that it was essential for one's economic base and social usefulness, but also that it served as a vehicle for the discharge of many other emotions.

Ginsburg,[2] in an article dealing with the effects of unemployment on the individual, makes clear that a person unable to find employment suffers a loss of sense of status and of identification with society. He speculates that we rely to a great extent on work as a source of self-evaluation and as a basis on which to pattern modes of adaptive behavior.

Hendrick[3] stated that work is the "expression of an instinct to master, whose goal is the control or alteration of environmental situations." He contrasted this drive to sexual pleasure, which he felt was primarily a discharge of tensions in the autonomic nervous system.

Lantos[4] saw work in terms of self-preservation. To quote her, "Work is related to self preservative instincts. Men do not work spontaneously. [The motive for work] is self preservation mediated by intelligence, reinforced by conscience, and aggression, which under conditions of civilization cannot find any direct outlet, becomes internalized and used by the superego to make the ego exert all its resources and submit to hardship and boredom. This internalized aggression is the ultimate guarantee of the maintenance of work."

Weber[5] characterized the so-called Protestant ethic as emphasizing the importance of "this world" and work as a "calling" with emphasis on industrious habits, punctuality, and a willingness to perform duties without special pay. Calvinism emphasized that one who labored earnestly, without complaint and with diligence, was doing God's work on earth. ". . . Faith had to be proved by its objective results in order to provide a firm foundation for the *certitudo salutis*. In practice, this means that God helps those who help themselves." The uncertainty among Calvinists as to whether one had been designated as one of the chosen could be allayed by the evidence of successful performance in the world via the appropriate material rewards of success. A counterpart occurs in Japanese culture according to De Vos,[6] who writes, "To be lazy is to injure the parents . . . and leads to intense guilt feelings."

The tendency to overwork probably is related to many of the qualities of personality noted by Friedman et al[7] in the type A personality with respect to greater proneness to coronary artery disease. Type A patients show an excessive sense of time urgency, pre-occupation with deadlines, and enhanced competitive drives.

The inability to enjoy holidays was described by Ferenczi,[8] who noted that many individuals were quite miserable on vacations or on Sundays, their days of rest from work. *Newsweek* (Sept 1, 1975, p 42) quotes an article by Susan Verman entitled "Why Women Can't Get Laid in San Francisco" as saying, "It's the straights who seem to be leery of sex. They drive themselves so hard during the day and then drink to get to sleep so they don't have any libido left at all." These statements echo those given by some patients: "I must remember to set aside some time to be spontaneous." "Fun is something you have to learn to do by working hard at it."

Szekely[9] believed that a drive to overwork (ie, to succeed) could be seen as a competition with an idealized version of one's father caused by an unresolved Oedipus complex.

Others have regarded work as what one must do to stay alive. Voltaire[10] expressed himself through *Candide* thus: "Work keeps at bay the great evils: Boredom, vice, and need." Mark Twain,[11] in *Tom*

Sawyer, expressed the view that "Work consists of whatever a body is *obliged* to do, and that play consists of whatever a body is not obliged to do." That the need may become a habit is expressed in the folk story of the man who worked hard in the mines all day to make money, to buy food, to build strength, so he could work hard in the mines all day.

More recently, a hippie patient wondered, "What's this hang-up people have about work? If we just shared everything, there wouldn't be all these problems of uptight adults and of having to work." Still another attitude toward work was expressed by Parkinson[12]. "Work expands so as to fill the time available for its completion," a remarkably perceptive view of the bureaucratic concept of toil.

ROLE OF CONSCIENCE

Most authors see the attitude toward work as stemming from the conscience and based on (1) a reaction against or an incorporation of parental and cultural attitudes, (2) a basis of self-evaluation, and (3) a convenient vehicle for displacement or sublimation of certain drives. Despite the complaints about the Protestant ethic and Puritan conscience, there are few articles that deal specifically with problems of overwork, in contrast to a large number dealing with inability or unwillingness to work. Either we are not as puritanical as most writers think, or else we are all so agreed on the inherent sinfulness of laziness that we overlook even the occasional evidences of overwork.

The cases described and listed illustrate the syndrome of overwork as it occurs in various types of personalities, with varied occupations, with a variety of diagnoses of varying degrees of severity, and with varied outcomes. In common, the patients exhibit problems in dealing with aggressive impulses and guilt feelings, they work in open-ended occupations (where each has his own conscience as the monitor that decides how much is enough), and they attempt to solve their life problems by excessive work done in a compulsive manner. Several were trying to meet current situations in a manner similar to that by which they had dealt with earlier life insecurities but where the old method was inappropriate for the new circumstances. Others had identified strongly with a demanding, unpleasable parent, making that person's demands a part of their own conscience and living a life subservient to this harsh, uncompromising part of themselves. Narcissistic injuries played a prominent part in the illness of several others, who were unable to accept the physical limitations of poor health or aging. In physicians, particularly, the need to be loved by everyone was a major component of the drive to overwork. Three of the physicians rationalized, "My patients need me; I know their cases better than anyone else." Fear of failure to live up to ideals and goals played a prominent part in all cases. In a few instances, a continuing need to compete, originally with a childhood rival, became a way of life. In addition, overwork may represent an effort to maintain a clear conscience by saying to the world, "See, I am blameless. I have done all that I could, even working to the edge of total exhaustion."

The overwork syndrome may mimic a number of other illnesses: anxiety neurosis, depression, myocardial infarction, organic brain syndromes, hypoglycemia, and thyroid deficiency, to name a few. It may lead, through self-treatment, to alcoholism or drug dependency. Diagnosis depends on a careful evaluation of the physical status of the patient and a history that includes attention to the evolution and progression of the symptoms and a consideration of the work attitudes and habits of the individual. Many persons are able to work equally long hours without becoming ill. Those who become ill are those who ignore their body's signals for rest, recuperation, and recreation. One must keep in mind that people differ individually in their amounts of available energy, recuperative powers, and in enjoyment of work. All these factors affect the development of the overwork syndrome.

Treatment depends on the assessment of the underlying causes. In severe cases, hospitalization and specialized treatment may be necessary. In mild cases, a vacation and counseling regarding future work vs recreation and rest may be all that is required. In any event, an evaluation of the patient's attitudes toward work is essential to avoid recurrences.

REFERENCES

1. Freud S: *Civilization and Its Discontents*, ed 21. London, Hogarth Press, 1961, pp 59–145.
2. Ginsburg SW: What unemployment does to people. *Am J Psychiatry* 99: 432–446, 1942.

3. Hendrick I: Work and the pleasure principle. *Psychoanal Q* 12: 311–329, 1943.

4. Lantos B: Metapsychological considerations in the concept of work. *Int. J Psychoanal* 33: 439–443, 1952.

5. Weber M: *The Protestant Ethic and the Spirit of Capitalism*, Parsons T (trans-ed). London, George Allen & Unwin Ltd, 1956, pp 114, 115.

6. De Vos G: The relation of guilt toward parents to achievement and arranged marriage among the Japanese. *Psychiatry* 23: 287–301, 1960.

7. Friedman M, Rosenman RH, Straus R, et al: The relationship of behavior pattern A to the state of coronary vasculature. *Am J Med* 44: 525–527, 1968.

8. Ferenczi S: Sunday neuroses, in Rickman J: *Further Contributions to the Theory and Technique of Psychoanalysis*, Suttie JI (trans-ed). New York, Basic Books Inc Publishers, 1953, pp 174–177.

9. Szekely L: Success, success neurosis and the self. *Br J Med Psychol* 33: 45–51, 1960.

10. Voltaire: *Candide*, chap 30.

11. Twain M: *Tom Sawyer*, chap 2.

12. Parkinson CN: *Parkinson's Law*. Boston, Houghton, Mifflin Co, 1957, p 2.

I'm a Doctor—
And a Drug Addict

Anonymous

A few of you may sympathize with me, but most of you probably think of drug abusers as human garbage. Until recently, I felt that way myself. The opinion formed in 1974 when, after graduating from medical school, I was briefly put in charge of a hospital's alcohol-detox unit. It seemed clear that my patients were just disgustingly weak-willed people who couldn't break the habit of dumping ethanol into their bodies.

Back then, the only drug I took was an occasional amphetamine to keep me alert on days after I'd moonlighted in the local emergency room. The long hours and chemical pep seemed justified by my $20,000 education debt, my impending marriage to a woman with two sons (ages 5 and 11 at the time), and by the fact that we'd soon move to Texas, where I was to begin a three-year pediatric residency paying $9,000 a year.

The Texas hospital had a rigorous teaching program, a heavy census, and a shortage of residents. Throughout 1975, I was on call every third night and usually couldn't sleep. Also, since my family was barely staying afloat financially, I spent weekends either moonlighting or on call. In order to maintain that brutal pace, I was taking 12½ mg of amphetamines every morning.

My family's allergies, aggravated by the Texas climate, forced me to hunt for another residency. None was available, but by the end of the year I landed a position with a group-practice clinic in a small Southern town. My colleagues—two GPs, two surgeons, and an OB man—would concentrate on the adults, while I took care of the pediatric patients.

I built up my new practice to 25 patients a day during 1976. Adding a generous salary to what I made by continuing to moonlight, I increased my annual take-home pay to $50,000. I also increased my daily amphetamine dose to 25 mg.

The use of stimulants hardly seemed cause for alarm. They made me talk faster than normal, but people at the clinic had never heard me talk any other way, and I always took the capsules at home. Serious physical addiction to amphetamines isn't supposed to be possible, so I didn't worry about periodically boosting the dosage to maintain the extra-energy effect.

By 1977, I'd purchased a nice home, repaid a substantial chunk of my school loan, and was seeing 35 patients a day. My morning intake of amphetamines had jumped to 37½ mg.

My wife, who's a medical lab technician, began expressing concern in early 1978. The drugs probably weren't good for me, she'd say, and what if the Drug Enforcement Administration were to question my need for so many diet pills? Convinced that I wasn't addicted, I told her I would quit taking the amphetamines during a forthcoming family vacation.

I tried to keep my promise. I stopped taking the drug, and almost immediately my energy level plummeted. I became a crabby, depressed s.o.b. who wanted only to lie in the hotel bed. When our boys popped open the door from their adjoining room to ask if I wanted to go swimming, I told them to leave me alone. When my wife asked if I'd like to take a walk on the beach at sunset, I told her to go by herself.

FROM DRUG TO DRUG

Two days off the stimulants, and I couldn't live with myself. I started taking an oral narcotic—one tablet three times a day—to smooth out my mood. It worked fine for a while. I became a good father and husband again, and the rest of the vacation went nicely without amphetamines.

I figured that I'd take the narcotic for a week or so until my energy returned, but I enjoyed the effect so much that I just kept taking it. Soon I reinstituted my amphetamine regimen, too.

Although it didn't seem very important at the time, I moved into the newly constructed pediatric wing of our clinic in October 1978. Instead of working closely with the other doctors, as I had been, I now saw them only when one of my patients needed referral to a surgeon. Rarely was anyone around of sufficient rank to question my behavior, and my behavior got worse.

The first narcotics prescription I'd written—for 50 tablets—lasted about a month. The exhilarating "rush" began to fade. I stepped up the dosage—one every four hours, one every three hours, one every two hours—until I couldn't get a buzz off a tablet an hour. Solution: Take two, or even three, at once.

By December 1978, I was downing 100 tablets every three days and writing prescriptions for them at all seven drugstores in town. Nevertheless, I wasn't entirely conscious of my addiction until I ran out of the drug one Sunday. I began having withdrawal symptoms and was scared to death. Somehow, I managed to survive until the next morning, then raced to a drugstore. I got there before the pharmacist and, when he arrived, I mumbled something about my back pain—"lumbar laminectomy, 1968." Feeling guilty and nervous as hell, I ordered a bottle of 100 tablets. He filled it without blinking an eye.

Even so, I worried about the DEA catching up with me and about how to get unhooked. The anxiety, combined with large doses of narcotics and amphetamines, was making me irritable. On the job at the clinic, I began to lose my cool.

One mother, for example, was supposed to bring in her son for a follow-up visit after she'd made a calendar showing the days on which the boy had soiled his pants. She brought him back, but without the calendar. I told her icily not to darken my doorway again unless she could follow instructions.

Word of my personality change must have been spread by the office staff, because one of the senior physicians called me into conference. What was bothering me? Why was I being such a bastard? Was I having problems at home? No, absolutely nothing was wrong, I insisted. At that, he let the matter drop.

A potential confrontation had been avoided, but the internal and external pressures to quit my habit were mounting. I talked it over with my wife, who was supportive yet worried. She knew I'd been taking narcotics but was floored when I told her how much. We agreed that I should spend a few days at home after Christmas and withdraw.

On the morning of Dec. 26, I stopped taking the drug. By the next day, though, my skin had become so hypersensitive that it would "crawl" in pain when touched—or at the mere thought of being touched. To end that horrible sensation, I began taking narcotics again. *How could I stop it*? The idea that I might not be able to quit was terrifying, yet I ordered another bottle from a wholesale house.

The problem was compounded a few days later, at the beginning of 1979, when pyloric spasms made it difficult to keep food down and midepigastric pain began waking me up at 3 a.m. I'd take some antacids, lie on the living room couch, hold my stomach, and try to sleep. The antacids didn't touch the pain. I went to my bag and pulled out the bottle of meperidine hydrochloride I'd carried ever since getting my DEA number in 1976. An injection of 100 mg did the trick.

On Jan. 23, our anniversary, my wife and I checked into a hotel, planning to spend a romantic evening together. We began the celebration by asking room service to send us a sumptuous meal. After eating, I went into the bathroom and threw up.

I continued the meperidine in conjunction with an ulcer medication only until the stomach pain resolved. Then I began wondering again how to get off the narcotic. If I confided in another doctor, I'd risk exposure, so that was out of the question.

A TRY AT SELF-TREATMENT

Already, my nurse at the clinic had caught on. After finding an empty narcotics bottle in the wastebasket, she asked: "Why are you using drugs? Don't you know that if you keep using them, you're going to hurt yourself? That you might even die?"

Nothing to be concerned about, I told her. I was about to go on a 10-day vacation, and when I returned I'd be drug-free.

I'd studied the narcotics section of a pharmacology textbook and learned that withdrawal couldn't kill me. I had also found out that the acute symptoms—such as crawling skin—would last only three or four days. Conclusion: By keeping myself heavily sedated for about 72 hours, I'd no longer be an addict.

My wife and I sent the boys to stay with their grandparents, then put the plan into effect. Quitting both the amphetamine and the narcotics, I took 200 mg of a barbiturate PO on a Friday night and fell asleep. When I woke up on Saturday, I took 25 mg of an antihistamine PO and 10 mg of a tranquilizer PO. The next time I regained consciousness, I took the barbiturate again. By alternating the drugs, I wouldn't overdose on the barbiturate.

For three days, my loving wife maintained a vigil at my side. She checked my pulse and blood pressure and tried to keep track of how many pills I took. She read books, watched television, and paced. Once in a while, she'd wake me up to ask if I was all right. "Leave me alone," I'd tell her. "I know what I'm doing."

And actually, it seemed as though I did. I returned to work chemically free in February. Elated at the success of my plan, I started a rough draft of a manuscript I hoped *Medical Economics* would print to show other addicted doctors how they, too, could get off drugs all by themselves.

Two weeks later, I got back on amphetamines again. Moonlighting, you see—I had to stay awake. Four weeks after the vacation, my daily dose had climbed to 50 mg. It held there through March and April. As far as anyone else knew, I appeared to have conquered addiction, but I put my manuscript into a folder and tossed it on a shelf.

FROM BAD TO WORSE

In May, one of my wife's close friends died, and so did her grandmother and my father. To top that off, our oldest son developed serious behavioral problems in school and told us he wanted to leave home. My wife entered a period of severe depression, while I secretly returned to narcotics.

In June, when my wife's depression had subsided, I let her know that I was back on narcotics. What I didn't share with her was that I had also become addicted to the meperidine.

At first, I'd rationalized that nightly 100 mg injections of the meperidine were necessary if I was to get any sleep. After all, the worries over family problems and the narcotics use—in addition to the wide-awake effect provided by amphetamines—were giving me insomnia. Within six weeks, though, I was shooting up 400 mg of the meperidine each morning, followed by 200 mg every two hours. And I was having difficulty finding a vein.

I'd lock myself in the office and probe my arms, legs, ankles, and feet for 10 minutes or more—often poking myself 30 times before locating a usable vessel. On one occasion, I hit an artery in my wrist. My hand turned glowing red and burned like fire. I seriously thought I was about to lose my hand, but after 30 minutes the pain passed.

More typically, my needle would eventually pierce its intended target, and then my mouth would become so dry that it was difficult to talk. Pure pleasure would surge through my bloodstream, I'd sweat profusely, and finally feel totally drained. It was chemical orgasm.

This became my routine: I'd see three or four patients, take a 30-minute break and shoot up, change my sweat-drenched scrub suit, see a few more patients, and shoot again.

The other clinic doctors were not aware of this activity, but my nurse quickly picked up on it and asked pointedly: "Why do you go into your office and lock the door all the time? You've never done that before."

Upset though she was, she covered for me. She cleaned up the blood on my desk and disposed of the syringes and empty meperidine bottles I threw into the trash. When I became slower and slower in the office and the waiting time for patients increased, she interceded with patients and staff members alike. The doctor isn't feeling good, she'd tell them, but she would keep the office open to make sure he saw everyone scheduled.

The other nurses and assistants weren't happy about working two hours longer than normal every day, but I was in no hurry to get home. I wanted to be with my drug, not my family. I put off going home until 9 or 10 p.m., then avoided the children altogether, spending much of my time in the bedroom or bathroom shooting up.

Initially, to hide my bruised and needlemarked arms from my wife, I wore a white coat home from the office and refused to take it off. She soon deduced the obvious and reacted predictably, however, throwing away any meperidine she could find.

Between my wife and nurse, nearly every move I made was subject to scrutiny. They compared notes over the phone each day, and both repeatedly asked me in plaintive voice, "How can you do this to yourself?"

Growing more secretive and remote, I started shooting up in bathrooms at the hospital, in restaurants, and in department stores. I also began doing something I'd never done before—lying to my wife.

She would catch me shooting up, and I'd promise to quit. In fact, I *would* withdraw for a couple of days at a time, but only to wait for the next meperidine shipment from the wholesale house. I'd know exactly when it was due, and I'd have my sleeve rolled up before I got the box open.

Surprisingly, my wife never threatened to leave me. Although I love her deeply, it wouldn't have made any difference to me if she'd walked out. An addict lets nothing come between himself and his drugs.

At work, of course, patients and their parents got in the way. I dreaded talking with them. If a mother started to ramble on with minor concerns about her kids, I'd cut her short and tell her to get to the point. Further, I used to receive about 20 calls a day from parents wanting to discuss their children's health problems. While on the meperidine, I returned only the most pressing calls. My nurse handled the rest as well as she could.

.

Reclusiveness was only one of a lengthening list of addiction symptoms that were becoming more difficult to conceal. My eyes had sunken, and my speech was slurred. I lost weight, my skin took on a leathery look, and I was chronically groggy. The rumor among patients and office staffers was that I'd turned into an alcoholic.

THE CRISIS STAGE

Clearly, the writing was on the wall. Having exhausted the veins in parts of my anatomy normally covered by clothing, I was forced to concoct excuses to account for the fresh injection sites and swelling on the dorsum of my hands. Scratched myself while picking blackberries, I was planning to tell the curious. But no one ever asked me.

On Friday, July 20, 1979, the crisis of my addiction began. My meperidine supply arrived at the clinic, but the wholesaler had neglected to include my name on the shipping label. Consequently, a part-time nurse opened the box and showed its contents to one of my colleagues. He brought the drug to me and said he'd like to have a talk with me on Saturday.

The following afternoon, as soon as I'd seen all my scheduled patients, I quickly left the clinic and avoided the showdown. I drove to an isolated, wooded area where roads had recently been graded for a new subdivision. There, I parked in a dead-end lovers' lane and stuck a butterfly tube in a vein. That way, I wouldn't have to keep jabbing myself with a needle. For the next four hours, I gave myself repeated shots of meperidine, lapsing unconscious after each injection.

When I walked in the door that evening, my wife was in tears. She'd sent the children on a bus to stay with their grandparents. Instead of being angry, however, she threw her arms around me and continued to cry. I started to cry, too. We spent the next three hours holding each other and sobbing.

It had finally dawned on me how much pain I'd been inflicting on my wife. I truly wanted to stop, and I was still convinced that I could quit on my own. If everyone would just get off my back, if the kids wouldn't fight so much, if I didn't have to work so hard—the old But/If Syndrome. Luckily, my wife knew more about addiction than I did.

She'd been on the phone trying to find out what to do. A psychiatric hospital had referred her to Ridgeview Institute near Atlanta, headquarters of Georgia's Disabled Doctors Program.[1] Through conversations with the director, my wife began to see the big difference between withdrawing from drugs and not wanting to use them anymore. She understood that I couldn't overcome the desire by myself, no matter how much I loved her or how hard I tried.

Despite her insights and arguments, though, I resisted the idea of entering a rehabilitation program. In response, without my knowing it, she enlisted my brother in the cause.

Sunday was my 30th birthday, and I spent most of it bolstering my determination to quit drugs. The only real causes for celebration were that I hadn't yet lost my license, my practice, my family, or my life.

On Monday, July 23, I stayed home from work and continued to withdraw. By evening, the urge to shoot had grown powerful. That's when my brother opened the front door and walked in—a total surprise for me! He'd left his pregnant wife and his job in California and had flown across the country to talk with me. His presence helped convey the gravity of my situation. After a couple of hours of discussion, I finally agreed to enter the Ridgeview Institute as a patient.

THE LONG ROAD BACK

Early Tuesday morning, at my request, I met with my colleagues from the clinic. In a hospital conference room, I let them know that I was addicted to meperidine, that I needed to do more than withdraw, and that I'd be leaving later in the day to start an extended course of treatment. I didn't know when or if I'd return to the clinic, so I advised them to find another pediatrician to replace me.

The other doctors were unanimously supportive. They said they'd hold a place open for me until I finished treatment and that I couldn't be replaced. I had trouble holding back the tears as I thanked them. We shook hands, then I left the room, went immediately to a drugstore, and bought another bottle of meperidine.

For two hours—while my wife and brother were anxiously waiting to begin the trip to Atlanta—I sat in the woods and shot up.

When I finally got home, they rushed along my packing and hustled me into the car. We hadn't gone 40 miles when I insisted on stopping at a drugstore. I bought more meperidine and used it at restaurants, rest stops, and hotels.

On Wednesday, July 25, my wife and brother dropped me off at the front door of Ridgeview Institute, where I said the hardest goodbye I've ever had to say. I was ashamed of myself and scared. My self-esteem was at its lowest. But worst of all, despite the love shown by my family, I felt *alone*. I didn't understand what was happening to me, or why.

Ridgeview took care of that. During the first few days, I was detoxed with the help of a tranquilizer. Then, as I became aware of the surroundings, my feelings about myself and my addiction changed.

I was lodged in a cottage with 30 other addicts and alcoholics, a third of whom were doctors, dentists, nurses, and veterinarians. All of a sudden, I didn't feel so alone. Most of the physicians and psychologists who examined me were also recovering addicts. I was treated like a person, not a junkie.

The big breakthrough for me came during a lecture on the disease concept of addiction. I learned that I didn't have a "bad habit" that stemmed from a weak will—after all, I'd survived the rigors of medical school. My primary symptom was uncontrollable drug use, and I could no more change that by myself than a diabetic could will his urine sugar to be negative. The speaker went on to cite numerous studies indicating that people can be genetically predisposed to drug addiction and that not everyone who abuses drugs becomes an addict. My self-esteem rose 1,000 percent after his lecture.

I've since realized that—while I may not have been responsible for my disease—I am responsible for my recovery. I'll always feel compelled to abuse drugs, so I'll have to control the urge by using the many non-chemical coping techniques learned in the Ridgeview program.

I've had some practice at using those skills already. After a month at the institute, I moved into a halfway house with four other doctors who were also recovering addicts. We lived together for two months and, whenever our individual efforts at self-control got shaky, we set aside our pride and relied upon one another for assistance. That's an important skill in itself.

Today, rather than return to my clinic practice, I've decided to serve the final two years of my pediatric residency at a university hospital. This won't be easy, and I'm somewhat apprehensive at the prospect. I still have debts to pay and a family to support, and the position pays only $14,000 a year. That means, despite the long hours at the hospital, I'll probably start moonlighting again. And when I suffer from fatigue, I'll be tempted by my prescription pad. But I won't be alone anymore. A network of addictionologists, therapists, and recovering addicts will be ready to help me out. All I'll have to do is to ask.

NOTE

1. See "Doctor Rehabilitation: Is It Working?" *Medical Economics*, Nov. 27, 1979. Ridgeview Institute is located at 3995 South Cobb Drive, Smyma, Ga. 30080. Phone: (404) 434–4567.

Residency Stress Leading to Suicide: A Mother's View

Erika H. Rosemark

My daughter's internship, characterized by 6 months of extreme stress and exhaustion, ended in her suicide at the age of 26. This is her story as related to me and some of her friends through correspondence and personal contact.

On July 2, 1983, I drove from my home in Sherman Oaks, California to visit our daughter, Barbara, who had started her internship three weeks earlier. She had found an apartment that she liked about a mile from the hospital and seemed pleased with the way things were shaping up. Although she knew that this was going to be a difficult year, she told me how much she liked being there. As we toured the area, she commented how the tree-lined streets, the green parks and bike paths appealed to her great love for the outdoors. "I'm fortunate to be here," she said. "This is one of the best internship programs in Family Practice in the country. I like the people and feel comfortable with their approach to the practice of medicine. I'm learning a lot."

Barbara had shown us the printed outline for her Orientation Week and I, too, was impressed with the amount of thoughtful planning that had been done to prepare these young doctors for this rigorous year at the University Medical Center. I came away from that visit feeling very positive about Barbara's year as an intern. She was enthusiastic about her work, and with what she was learning, was near old friends and finding new ones. She loved her new surroundings.

The only thing that concerned me was that when she added up the number of hours she had worked that week, it totaled one hundred and eight. "What are they trying to do to you?" I asked in dismay. Now, after the loss of my only daughter, I ask the same question. Clearly, changes must be made now, before another valuable human life is lost.

BACKGROUND

Barbara was born in Los Angeles in 1957 and grew up in Sherman Oaks. Her family consisted of her father, an insurance agent and broker, her mother, an early childhood educator, and her older brother, now a physicist in medicine. Barbara's autobiographical sketch, prepared for her residency application, summarizes highlights of her life.

My brother and I were very much influenced by my parents and their values. My father, born to two immigrant parents, was the first in his family to go to college, and once there a new world opened up to him. He was excited about learning and continues to be a voracious reader. I found his enthusiasm to be contagious.

My mother's influence was more people-oriented. She was raised in Germany, where my grandmother practiced psychiatry and my grandfather was an internist. These grandparents instilled in my mother a concern for others, which she, in turn, passed on to me. My mother has worked in early childhood education most of her life. Whenever a child in her school was having problems, she worked intensively with the child and family. Through her shared experiences she gave me an understanding of family dynamics.

Since many of my relatives live in Europe, I travelled a great deal during my childhood. Until I entered college in 1975, I spent every third summer in Hamburg, Germany. This gave me an appreciation of many customs, languages, and values.

Going through the public schools in Van Nuys, California was interesting, because the area includes the well-to-do hills of Sherman Oaks as well as the barrio of Van Nuys. There I learned to deal with a varied cross-section of class mates. I worked hard in school and I did well in all my classes. What I enjoyed most were independent projects where I had to use some imagination or dig through references. At some point during high school, I began to consider medicine as a possible goal for the future.

For an undergraduate university, I chose M.I.T., because it encouraged independent study and learning by practical experience. We were taught what had been discovered in the past through experimentation and how to design experiments of our own. I concentrated my studies on two of my greatest interests:

biology and architecture. I enjoyed the variety this gave to my schedule. I also rowed on the Women's Crew Team and fixed houses for low-income families as a member of a service fraternity. During these years I worked on two projects in medical research and spent two summers as a volunteer in pediatric intervention programs at UCLA and Cedars-Sinai Hospitals. These experiences confirmed my interest in becoming a physician.

I moved back to Los Angeles in 1979 to attend the U.S.C. School of Medicine. Medical school was an experience of total immersion. We learned so much so quickly over the first two years. In the clinical years all that classroom material was put to use as we began to deal with pediatric and adult patients. I enjoy the detective work that goes on in making a diagnosis. I plan to educate my patients and their families each step of the way to counteract their fears of the unknown and to encourage them to become actively involved in their own health care. Family Practice is the field I have chosen, because it will enable me to practice preventative medicine and to work with patients of all ages.

INTERNSHIP EXPERIENCES

As Barbara began her internship, her first two rotations seemed to go well. She worked in ENT four weeks (6–23 to 7–19) and was on-call every third night. During the next month (7–20 to 8–16) she worked in Family Practice and received intensive first aid training.

Barbara's problems began with her next rotation in Ob-Gyn (8–17 to 9–13). She worked hard doing what she thought needed to be done, but was not clear what was expected of her. At this time signs of physical exhaustion began to show up. She developed cellulitis and food poisoning, but kept on working. On the last day of her Ob-Gyn rotation (9–13) Barbara phoned me crying and very upset. A woman resident had told her that she had not done a good job and had not kept up with the other interns. Barbara pointed out that she was the only Family Practice intern on the rotation (the rest were from the Department of Ob-Gyn) and had not been told what to do.

The next day, which was supposed to be the first day of her vacation, she phoned again, saying that she had been crying all night and day and found it difficult to concentrate on work. She said that she felt emotionally worn out, but could not come home because she was left with many discharge summaries to complete.

After finishing her work, Barbara spent the remaining vacation time visiting friends and relatives on the East Coast and having a good time. Returning to her internship, she began a NICU rotation (10–12) which turned out to be another very stressful time for her. Her reactions at this time are conveyed in a letter written to a friend (11–11).

Within the past 48 hours my environment has made several radical shifts and I'm not sure I have my bearings yet. I finally finished up at the NICU. Then spent one day running errands, washing clothes, cleaning up my apartment, and taking a friend to the airport. The next morning I packed up my car, including bicycle and cross-country skis, and headed up north for my next rotation, with my fingers crossed that my car would make it all the way up the 160 mile drive.

Throughout this time I just felt "out of it," half comatose. I keep having flashbacks to those babies, all lined up in a row, in their radiant open warmers—IV's going into their scalps, another line going into their umbilicus, with a tube down their throats connected to the respirator. Then to keep down evaporative loss of fluids, these little beings, looking more like rat pups than human babies, are covered in saran wrap. Now imagine the sounds in the room. Each bedside gadget has a different alarm. The heart-rate monitor has a quick repetitive high-pitched whistle, which goes off about as often from leads coming loose as it does from a true slowed heart rate. The IV's are on electric pumps which beep, if their flow is interrupted. The temperature probe on each baby buzzes, if the baby gets too hot or too cold. In the background there is usually radio music, respirator noises, and nurses calling out the latest blood gas results.

By the time I reached my destination, my eyes felt very tired and everything looked blurry. My eyes seem to have deteriorated over the past month. Either that or I haven't been outside enough to remember that my vision at far distances is blurred. Time to get a new pair of glasses.

Unfortunately, the first task I had to face after arriving was an "in-house exam". Every year they give us this six-hour multiple-choice exam as preparation for the Family Practice Specialty Boards, so they can see how much we have to improve to pass the real thing. Sigh! One more hoop to jump through. One more day of realizing how much I don't know and how much I'll probably never know, or be able to remember. That's one thing I find very depressing about medicine—there is always too much to know. Maybe later on, when I've had more experience, I'll reach a point at which I'm satisfied with what I know, but I'm not there yet.

I also noticed on arriving at this community hospital that I became very conscious of being a woman. One of the doctors from the Family Practice Clinic was introducing me to various people in the cafeteria. "This is Barbara," he said to one nurse. "She'll be up here next year, so you'll just have to get used to dealing with women." The nurse looked perplexed. "I know how to deal with women," she replied. I felt like saying, "It's this doctor's problem." I hope situations like this will not distract me from my work. Guess that's the price I pay for being the first woman in this particular program.

At the Affiliated Hospital, Barbara found her new adjustment difficult. When I asked her how things were going, she replied, "Not the greatest. I feel tired and stressed and very scared! This is not a teaching hospital, and they have a different way of practicing medicine. They don't ask for tests before making a diagnosis, and I'm finding that hard to deal with. The nurses are not used to working with new interns, and when I do things less than perfectly, they exchange critical looks. But most of all I feel unsupported when I'm left totally alone with the patients in the hospital at night. That responsibility terrifies me!"

Toward the end of this rotation, Barbara came home for Thanksgiving. It was so good to have her home and have a chance to spoil her a bit. She, too, enjoyed being with us, and seeing her friends, but from time to time I saw glimpses of her extreme exhaustion and sense of despair.

Sunday night came and went much too soon, and Barbara did not want to go back. I tried to find out if there was someone she could talk to about all these overwhelming experiences. I hated to see her go back with all these problems unresolved.

During the next few days we called each other, as usual, and Barbara sounded very depressed. When I asked her what she was doing about this, she replied that she had made an appointment with a psychologist. A few days later she said that she had seen him but it was not very helpful. "I'm panicking!" she said. "I find it hard to face new situations over and over again! I want to come home and have someone take care of me!"

Naturally I was greatly alarmed. I called a faculty member, who had been Barbara's advisor in medical school, and told him what was happening. This doctor was very understanding and offered to call the physician in charge of Barbara's program to make him aware of the situation.

Barbara talked with the Director of her residency program (12–19) and was referred to a clinical psychologist for help, and to a third-year resident who had encountered some of the same problems earlier. The Director also reviewed her evaluations with her and pointed out that she had done some outstanding work. But Barbara felt that she was not doing well and could not accept positive feedback. They discussed the possibility of a leave of absence. At this point, however, Barbara apparently was beyond the point of being able to reach out for the help that she needed.

During the next few days she deteriorated rapidly. Feeling powerless and so far away, I hoped that she could be hospitalized and medicated under the care of a psychiatrist. All of us at home felt desperate and totally helpless. When she told us that she could not function at work and was hiding at the hospital, we suggested that she ask for a leave of absence and come home. On December 22, she did ask for a leave and told us that she would think about coming home. From then on it was very difficult to reach her; she was either out or did not answer the phone. When I finally connected with her (12–23) she seemed to have trouble thinking and talking; her voice would fade away. Again I asked her to come home or if she wanted me to come up to be with her. At one point she said that she would try to get a flight home, but later said that she was not feeling well.

The last person to speak with Barbara was her brother, Peter. She called him at 1 p.m. on Christmas Eve and when asked if he could come up to be with her, she replied, "Oh another one who wants to come up here." He felt as if he had said the wrong thing.

At this point we lost all contact with Barbara. The Director of her program went to her apartment the day after Christmas and found that Barbara and her car were gone. He notified the police and she was declared a missing person. A very dedicated woman detective from the Campus Police Department and many of Barbara's close friends began an exhaustive search. Not until January 25, 1984 was Barbara's car found abandoned at a steep cliff overlooking the ocean.

The following note, written in November 1983, was later found in Barbara's apartment:

> I get to such depths of sadness when I've been on call. Usually it happens just after getting home. That's when I realize that I haven't been leading a life away from the hospital. No time. Piles of dirty clothes. Stacks of magazines and several days' mail on the table not yet opened. Bills collecting, unpaid for unknown lengths of time. Unread newspapers—depressing to even see, because they are a sign of how much I don't know about what has been happening in the world beyond the third floor of the medical center. That is my world now.

I get jealous of the nurses and techs and clerks who can go home after their eight hours. On call I see five changes of personnel before opening that door to my home.

I see the women coming in to see their babies in the hospital. They hold them and look into the baby's face with such adoring eyes. Sometimes a husband is there by their side and those eyes shift from father to baby with the same delight. I suppose I'm viewed to be in a better position than those parents, who have a child sick in the hospital. After all, I'm young, not sick, and pursuing my "challenging career." But when I look at these couples, I feel such emptiness. What am I giving up to devote so much of myself to my work? I want to be the one with those delighted eyes, with one finger tightly grasped by a tiny little hand. I want to be the one beaming across to the man at my side with eyes that say, "Look at this miracle we've made," without speaking a word.

After call everything upsets me. I try to compress a few days' needs for self-care and expression and communication into a few hours. Then I get angry, because that is not possible. Something always falls short, leaving me unsatisfied. I can't even say that I hate this way of living, because it is *not* living. I don't have a life now. It's out on lease.

CONCLUSION

What can we learn from Barbara's experience? What changes in the training program can be implemented now to spare future interns such emotionally disabling experiences?

In the hope that young physicians of the future may thrive in their training environment rather than being emotionally impaired by it, I offer this list of recommendations:

1. Require reasonable working hours. Expecting doctors to work 36 hours at a stretch and 100 hours or more per week may endanger their lives and well-being as well as minimize their effectiveness with patients.
2. Provide emotional support, such as weekly rap groups, where interns can talk about their stressful experiences and get support from each other and from more experienced doctors.
3. Provide clear guidelines before interns begin each new rotation so that they will know what is expected.

4. Avoid leaving new and inexperienced physicians feeling that they are without backup support; when they ask for help, provide appropriate support.
5. Provide encouragement and positive feedback throughout the entire training period. Offer positive guidance instead of blaming for mistakes.
6. Provide extra-close supervision and follow-up for interns who may be in distress. Sleep-deprived and under intense pressure, these trainees are clearly at risk and need protection.

In a profession whose goal is to promote health and well-being, it is puzzling to find that the training process sometimes disregards factors that contribute to the maintenance of physical and emotional health. How can physicians, whose own health and happiness is being ignored, adequately treat their patients with compassion and concern?

Preventing Physician Suicide: The Role of Family, Colleagues, and Organized Medicine

Douglas A. Sargent, Viggo W. Jensen, Thomas A. Petty, and Herbert Raskin

A former medical school classmate had killed herself. The same day I learned of her death, I also had a frustrating discussion with an insurance man who maintained that doctors would not buy adequate coverage for mental disorders because of the cost. I reasoned that it is not sensible to offer skimpy policies to doctors who both need and could afford better. He was adamant. "They won't sell," he said.

These events reminded me of other doctors I had known who had killed themselves. One, a friend, came to mind. For several years, rumors had been circulating about this friend's failing stability. Suicide seemed likely. Other psychiatrists had heard these reports and we discussed what might be done to help him, but we came to no satisfactory conclusion. Within a year, our failing friend had killed himself.

Why does the medical profession not do a better job of preventing suicide among its members than it does? This question prompted the following exploration (D.A.S.).

PREVALENCE

Suicide accounts for a remarkable number of deaths among physicians.[1,2] Doctors kill themselves at a rate equivalent to one medical school class each year. The tip of this statistical iceberg is visible almost every week in the obituary pages of *JAMA*.

Individual and group psychodynamics involving the doctor's professional and personal life make the recognition and effective treatment of potential suicide difficult. Furthermore, organized medicine has done little to overcome the problems arising from these psychodynamics. The care of our disturbed colleagues falls most heavily on psychiatrists, whose work will be facilitated by an understanding of these dynamics.

RECOGNIZING SUICIDAL PHYSICIANS

Impending suicide can be detected easily by anyone with no reason to conceal the signs from himself. The presuicidal physician usually comes from a disturbed family, had a "barren childhood," was a good student, and often is an older doctor, a psychiatrist, or a woman.[1-3] Single or unhappily married, the doctor abuses alcohol and is depressed, a condition to which doctors are prone.[4,5]

Suicidal dynamics begin with a narcissistic injury: failing health, marriage or practice, aging, retirement. Depression follows, often with suicidal thoughts; this easily deteriorates into overt self-destruction. The failing physician rationalizes signs of decompensation as the results of overwork and may seek relief in self-medication. He may resist getting professional help, instead increasing his already-frantic pace to conceal signs of deterioration. A person close to the doctor may be forced to become a rescuer, responding to the cries for help, which by now may be thinly disguised acts demonstrating suicidal intent.[6,7]

BARRIERS TO RECOGNITION

One would expect the sick doctor to have easy access to the professional attention of colleagues and the personal concern of family. However true this may be for other disorders, too often a psychological barrier is interposed between the depressed, suicidal doctor and these health resources, a barrier rooted in the minds of the doctor, family, and colleagues.[6]

Physician's Psychological Barrier

Doctors tend to regard personal illness as weakness, a narcissistic injury which triggers defensive psychic regression and impairs reality-appreciation, allowing the doctor to deny a suicidal danger that would be quickly detected in a patient. This denial is often supported by the doctor's fantasy that he or she is a miraculous healer, immune to disease. The tragic consequences of such denial and fantasy are illustrated in the following description.

The Doctor Who Worked Himself to Death

A busy general practitioner had surgical privileges withdrawn suddenly at the age of 60 years. Angry and indignant, he resigned from the hospital staff and threw himself into his other work. He bought a Rolls Royce, attired himself in morning clothes and top hat, and made house calls on his startled patients.

He was increasingly irritable during the day and restless at night, retiring late and sleeping for only a few hours after heavy sedation. He often saw 90 office-patients daily. He requested complicated surgical trays for procedures that were strange to his office.

Alarmed by these attempts at "professional suicide," his wife urged the doctor to consult a psychiatrist. He rejected this suggestion. She then conspired with a psychiatrist-friend of her husband to get him attention surreptitiously. By prearrangement, the psychiatrist called the doctor several nights a week for a friendly chat. With the wife's clever staging, the doctor was always home to receive the calls, and the plan was a partial success for a year. With his support, he became less irritable and stopped losing weight. But the shortcomings of the arrangement were obvious. He continued his crushing schedule of work. Shortly after the first anniversary of the doctor's resignation from the hospital, and following a night of sleepless agitation, he had a massive coronary occlusion and died.

To understand this tragic progression, we must look beyond the doctor's individual dynamics to the family, starting with the spouse.

Barrier in the Spouse

Frequently, a doctor's wife has married a god-like figure with whom she can establish a child-parent relationship. (Our data only cover doctors' wives. The portrait of the woman doctor's husband awaits further study.) The doctor is more worshipped than loved. The wife makes "sacrifices," rationalizing that the doctor's work demands them. When he becomes depressed, his wife may react with contempt at this evidence of "weakness." Resentment at the doctor's preoccupation with patients and neglect of the family surfaces when he becomes depressed, blocking her recognition of impending suicide. There is a strongly implied "now it is my turn to be taken care of" in the wife's failure to recognize signs of the doctor's deterioration. In exchange for the "advantages" of marriage to a god, the wife often becomes a superwife, protecting the doctor from distractions so that he might devote himself to medicine. This role may hamper treatment of the suicidal physician, as illustrated by the wife of the doctor who worked himself to death.

> The doctor's wife was a resourceful woman who had helped put her husband through medical school. She had helped to manage his practice and had buffered him from all nonprofessional demands. Sometimes she had exercised her judgment without informing him. Typically, she never told her husband of the conspiracy with his psychiatrist-friend, explaining only that they were concerned about him. She was so sure of her judgment that she dismissed the dangers of this deception until it was too late.

Family's Psychological Barrier

A doctor's family may deny his illness, impending suicide, or symbolic pleas for help. A wife, by organizing the family's life around the doctor's needs, may provoke the children's resentment of him. The busy doctor may carry his medical demeanor home, issuing "doctor's orders" to the family when reasonable parental concern is required. The children's complaints may be stifled by the weight of their father's medical duties.

Thus, out of revenge for past hurts and a need to preserve the doctor's "omnipotence," the family may unconsciously encourage the doctor to act out this fantasy, intensifying the danger of suicide. The potential rescuer selected by the suicidal doctor will likely be one of these ambivalent family members.[6] The rescuer who fails will be made to feel a murderer. Often, this dilemma only provokes abhorrence and denial of the suicidal danger.

Barrier in Colleagues

Colleagues often react to signs of depression in a doctor with annoyance and denial of what seems a "weakness" in one of their supposedly invulnerable band. A colleague's wish to help the sick doctor may conflict with competitive impulses or with feelings of aversion, having been antagonized by the doctor's "I-don't-need-anyone" attitude. Also, handling suicidal tendencies in a fellow physician is a grave responsibility that colleagues may wish to avoid.

PROBLEMS OF TREATMENT

The depressed doctor needs someone to help him consult a psychiatrist. The difficulty physicians have in admitting illness requires this to be done with the utmost concern for his self-respect. An aggressive confrontation may precipitate suicide. Informal discussion, however, may gain the doctor's cooperation, because he is relieved that he no longer has to cope with the problem alone.

Often by the time the doctor reaches treatment, family and friends have been alienated, funds are gone, and medical insurance does not cover the treatment needed. Inadequate insurance increases the reluctance to seek treatment. Depressed doctors are especially loathe to accept "professional courtesy."

The doctor may try to protect an already-bruised pride by choosing a therapist who can be misled or controlled. The spouse may have to help correct this evasion. Or the doctor may subtly influence the diagnosis and modify the recommendation by withholding pertinent information. The spouse may have to give supplemental information over the doctor's objection. The doctor may resist an emotional relationship, or transference, to a fellow physician. Such resistance may originate in guilt over childhood "doctor games" of sexual exploration.[8] The spouse's presence dilutes this transference relationship and guilt and promotes the therapeutic relationship.

We do not recommend that the doctor should be treated like any other patient.[1] We advocate an attitude of collegial regard, which permits the doctor to sustain an already fragile self-respect. The doctor's cooperation, which may depend on this attitude, is vital, because outpatient treatment may be the only kind the doctor will accept. The psychiatrist must also be alert to the doctor's tendency to shift the responsibility for managing his practice onto the spouse. The spouse must be helped to stay well clear of medical responsibilities. However, if the spouse can be relied on to assume some responsibilities, she may help by screening calls for a doctor who has become unable to resist the demands of importunate patients and by scheduling patients if the doctor's time sense has become disrupted.

These steps help to buoy up a frail but salvageable doctor. It is crucial, however, to help the doctor recognize when he should not practice. He may have unwarranted confidence in his abilities and may need help to face his diminished capacities. The psychiatrist's advice alone may not reconcile the doctor to this limitation. The family may have to help. A family therapy format may be useful for this phase.

Contamination of the treatment by the therapist's own unconscious attitudes is a particular concern when the patient is also a doctor. The fear expressed by Pollack and Battle, "If we (the doctor and the psychiatrist) are alike in so many other ways, could we be alike in being mentally ill?"[9] may cause mishandling of the doctor's illness.

COMMENT

Awareness of the barriers we have described is vital to effective intervention and treatment. Overcoming them will require dedication and tact, qualities not always conspicuous in our peer relationships. It is well to remind ourselves that *primum non nocere* should guide us in dealing not only with our patients but also with our fellow doctor who is impaired.

REFERENCES

1. Waring E: Psychiatric illness in physicians: A review. *Compr Psychiatry* 15: 519–530, 1974.

2. Ross M: Suicide among physicians. *Psychiatry Med* 2: 189–198, 1971.

3. Pasnau R, Russell A: Psychiatric resident suicide: An analysis of five cases. *Am J Psychiatry* 132: 402–406, 1975.

4. Stecker E, Appel K, Palmer H, et al: Psychiatric studies in medical education: II. Neurotic trends in senior medical students. *Am J Psychiatry* 92: 937–958, 1936.

5. Pitts F, Winokur G, Steward M: Psychiatric syndromes, anxiety symptoms, and response to stress in medical students. *Am J Psychiatry* 118: 833–840, 1961.

6. Jensen V, Petty T: The fantasy of being rescued in suicide. *Psychoanal Q* 27: 327–339, 1958.

7. Schneideman E, Farberow N: *Clues to suicide.* New York, McGraw-Hill Book Co, 1957.

8. Marmor J: The feeling of superiority: An occupational hazard in the practice of psychotherapy. *Am J Psychiatry* 110: 370–376, 1953.

9. Pollack IW, Battle WC: Studies of the special patient. *Arch Gen Psychiatry* 9: 344–355, 1963.

10. Simmel E: The doctor game, illness, and the profession of medicine. *Psychoanal Reader* 1: 291–305, 1948.

When Doctors Fail to Care for Themselves: Adaptation of a Lecture

George E. Vaillant

Psychiatry 700A. (Behavioral Science in Medicine) is a course at Harvard Medical School designed to sensitize medical students to the importance of self-awareness, and to decrease the distance between them and the patients they see. The concluding lecture in this course was given by George E. Vaillant, who outlines defense mechanisms used by physicians, as well as the risks of those mechanisms.

Today, to pull together the six sections of this course, I need to synthesize aggression, drinking, drug abuse, anxiety, inheritance, and attachment. I'm going to do it the way a lot of teaching and learning is done in medical school: each upon each—as our laboratory diagnosis teacher used to say. That's how you pass your first nasogastric tube, and how you draw your first blood. So today I'm going to demonstrate the relevance to doctors, to you, of what you've been learning.

One purpose of a psychiatry course in medical school is to teach you to be wise and to have as much sense about human affairs as your grandparents: to grow old before your time. What you're really trying to learn from psychiatry, then, is to be rational in the face of irrational feelings and behavior—in the face of unreason.

I'd like to introduce you to the relevance of such unreason with two recent letters from members of the Harvard Medical School class of '67 to the *Alumni Bulletin*:

> It is an immensely sobering and painful thought to realize that out of my medical school class—a cohort of people in their late thirties—we have already lost six of our members, two through acts of God, one uncertain, and three quite definitely by their own hands. I fear that this is no more than one of the painful realities of life in an unbelievably demanding profession. Yet, I feel that we do not—as a group or profession—pay sufficient attention to this

factor in our lives. It provokes large numbers of reflections concerning mortality, stress, and the ability to help our colleagues when they need it, and similarly unseasonal but powerful reflections.

The other letter observes:

> The tragic death of John brings to six the members of my class who have died. Five have died at least in part because of maladaptive lifestyles. This death rate seems excessive since most members of the class of '67 are forty or under. Is there a problem with who is selected for Harvard or with the education experience or with career expectations? Does Harvard pay enough attention to teaching students and alumni how to cope with stress?

I have also seen unreason in the results of a long-range study which has followed a group of 268 men from college—before it was clear which of them might become physicians—to their sixth decade. The men were chosen in their sophomore year, out of classes from 1939 to 1944, for their academic, physical, and mental health. Forty-six of them became doctors. By the time they were fifty, drug use (regular use of tranquilizers or intermittant use of sleeping pills, amphetamines, and minor tranquilizers) was twice as great for the doctors as for the controls. Drug abuse (dependence on alcohol or drugs which damages a life, both occupationally and socially) was even more prevalent among the doctors: nine percent of the physicians versus one percent of the controls.

One of the physicians allowed diagnostic burholes to be drilled into his skull after developing nystagmus, ataxia, slurred speech, and seizures. Certainly one possible diagnosis would have been brain tumor. A few months after the holes were drilled his doctor was smart enough to test his blood for barbiturates, and only then discovered that his doctor-patient had been abusing sedatives for several years. The doctor-patient had denied it; his wife had denied it; the medical profession had denied it—yet it is sort of irrational to let people drill holes in your head.

The physicians in the long-range study also had a somewhat higher rate of unstable marriages. One marriage deteriorated to the point that the physician moved to the basement of his home. He prided himself on restraining his anger, asserting that the only thing that annoyed him about his wife was that she sometimes talked too long on the phone. He contemplated suicide, but fortunately had a good doctor who suggested that he see a psychiatrist. The doctor-patient explained that he was too busy to do anything like that. His physician asked, "Look, if a patient of yours came to you with this kind of a story, what would you tell the patient to do?" The potentially suicidal doctor got the message.

One of the advantages of following college sophomores into their sixth decade is that you can see things develop over time. One of our evaluation techniques was to use a blind rater—on the basis of ratings at eighteen—to select the sixteen "best" childhoods of those who became physicians and the thirteen bleakest. We found that drug use among physicians with the best childhoods was very similar to drug use among the controls. But the doctors with the worst childhoods later practiced an enormous amount of self-medication. This does not mean that medical school admissions committees should not admit people with unhappy childhoods. Some of the very finest physicians—the ones whom you would want as your own—are doctors who have had painful childhoods. Empathy is often learned the hard way. My point is that such individuals need to receive as well as give care.

I was asked recently by a lawyer to explain the term "impaired physician." My answer was that an impaired physician is really a code word which refers to the countertransference problems that hospital administrators and department chairmen and presidents of hospital boards have toward physicians who are in pain, and who misuse drugs, and who suffer psychiatric illness. Those with the countertransference problem initially tend to deny that anything is wrong, and then to feel anger at the impaired physician; they may even convince themselves that the physican has done something wrong.

At a great teaching hospital, for example, a resident made a suicide attempt during a period of crisis. A week later the resident was fired. In the same hospital, house officers who were seen crying in the pediatric intensive care unit were sent to the psychiatrist, as if there were something wrong with them. Another teaching hospital has physicians on the staff who in the past have abused opiates. Although the usual protocol would be compulsory urine monitoring, there is still no provision in that hospital for such testing. Yet the idea of a hospital not being able to test, for instance, the urine of diabetic physicians is inconceivable.

These stories seem inhumane, and yet they come from reasonable hospitals and reasonable people. They are the result of doctors failing to care for both doctors and themselves as they would other patients. I can only explain it by the psychoanalytic term, counter-transference.

Let's turn now to the coping strategies of physicians—unconscious adaptive styles that in psychoanalytic argot are sometimes called ego mechanisms of defense. There are four such mechanisms that doctors tend to use more than other people. Under stress, they can be used maladaptively; when well used, they enhance effective functioning—like clotting mechanisms in the body, or callus formation.

The first defense is altruism: doing unto others as you would want others to do unto you, with the important proviso that you get paid for it: for example, the surgeon who nobly gets up at three in the morning for a patient gets to drive home in a Ferrari. Giving unto others only becomes a strain when you're giving more than you yourself receive. One physician, from another study of physician-addicts, never really achieved altruism. Instead he used to comfort himself by inducing ravenous hunger through self-injected insulin and then consuming a gallon of ice-cream. He later substituted narcotics as a more efficient form of solace. Treated for his narcotic addiction, he developed a habit of drinking a gallon of milk a day.

Altruism is a neat defense; it didn't do Schweitzer any harm at all. But it's important to realize that it can put people at homeostatic risk. You've got to have as much coming into a system as you give out or you're in trouble.

The second defense that doctors use more than others is reaction formation. That is doing the very opposite, with passion, of what you would really like to do. For example, consider the cigarette addict who throws away his cigarettes and then points at ashtrays and says, "Yuck, a disgusting habit," when he is just dying to have one. Reaction formation in doctors is most dramatic in the area of dependency. According to the results of the Terman Study—a random sample of 1,528 individuals in California with IQ's over 140—people who go into medicine are more dependent than those who go into other professions.

It's one of the interesting things about medicine: we like taking care of other people because we are dependent, yet we tend to keep our dependency needs secret from ourselves. One way of doing so is to say when we get sick, "Gee, I couldn't possibly bother Dr. Jones. If I went to see him, it would disturb him. I know how hard he works, and besides, if I saw him there would be no fee," rather than thinking, "Neat: if I get sick, I can go to Dr. Jones, and it won't even cost me anything."

Reaction formation can go to extremes. One doctor drove seventy miles from Vermont to see me. He described a habit of injecting narcotics into his thigh with unsterile technique while driving to work at high speeds on the superhighway. Yet even then he wanted to deny the problem. In the course of the consultation he told me, with tears streaming down his face, that he wasn't depressed and didn't need help.

I'll give you an example of reaction formation that's closer to home. When I was in medical school we had to go to the health services for a physical exam. Down the hall was a sign that said 'Dr. Bojar', and people were sitting outside his office. I knew that he was the school psychiatrist. I thought, those poor bastards—having to be humiliated and subjected to this terrible thing of going to see Doctor Bojar: the name still conjures up a certain amount of horror.

A few years later, I was the psychiatrist to the Tufts medical students. I thought it was a neat job: I was a splendid fellow, and the students were lucky to see me because it didn't cost them anything. The sensible students came to see me when they had troubles, and the ones who didn't were dumb. And I never made the connection, as to what in God's name was going on—that I would be perfectly willing to accept other people's dependency, while the thought of ever using one of those people myself was a fate worse than death.

The third defence mechanism physicians use is to turn the other cheek. Remember, turning the other cheek is tricky; the fact that it's called passive aggression is no accident. But it's a reinforcing way to express aggression, because society loves a martyr: people want their kindly G.P. to come through the snow to see them at three in the morning.

The mother of one of the physicians in the longitudinal study said that when her children were two, she "used to give them switches and have them switch themselves when they were naughty." This is a rather extreme way of illustrating how some physicians are socialized way before they get to medical school. Being a martyr isn't something that you necessarily learn here; it isn't something that is done to you by these marble buildings. Of course it's important in medicine not to show anger towards your patients. But it's an occupational hazard that one absorbs a great deal of anger and doesn't have any terribly good place to put it. Doctors need to develop healthy outlets for anger.

The fourth defense, to which I've already alluded in several ways, is dissociation, or neurotic denial. Dissociation is the feeling I had all through my internship, that only a silver bacillus could catch me—I've never believed in the germ theory with regard to myself.

Dissociation, like the other defenses, can go to extraordinary extremes. One of my colleagues, to help me illustrate the denial used by doctors, gave his case history of cancer to a Tufts class. He told an incredible saga of ignoring a growing exhaustion, until his wife found him asleep on the floor one morning and insisted that he see a doctor. His hematocrit showed that he had bled out half of his blood volume: he had intestinal cancer, and was operated on. He presented himself to the class as a five-year cure. He said, "It's neat, you know, having had cancer the way I have, because I've had one cancer and that means I won't get another and I can go on smoking."

That attitude just doesn't make sense. When marathon runners get tired, they look upon sleep and fatigue as friends. They don't try to stamp them out. What do you do when you have a patient in the hospital with pneumonia or an F.U.O.? You don't pour aspirin down his throat. You get a chart, and you chart the fever, and you use the fever as some index of what is going on, as your friend. What do doctors do when they have trouble sleeping or get tired? They take pills like Quaalude and Dexamil to stamp out such symptoms, rather than seeing the symptoms as signs they may need help.

What are the rules for dealing with all of this? First, you should realize that although altruism is a super defense, you should make sure that when you give to others, you're also given to. It doesn't mean that your childhood has to have been perfect—your past isn't inevitably going to follow you around all your life—but it is important that you make sure you're cared for now.

Next, find ways of expressing anger. They can be perfectly ingenious; I know you get a little practice in the second and fourth-year shows by evening the score with some of the people here who have made your lives miserable.

The last rule is really the most important, and if this is the only thing you take away with you from this class, it will be worth the effort. Never, as long as you live, take a pill that you have prescribed for yourself. Instead, ask a colleague to write the prescription. Under *no* circumstances should you ever self-medicate your central nervous system, and the reason is terribly simple: all pills that help the brain feel better work, in part, because they are symbols of another person caring for you. If you do it for yourself, it's like trying to tickle yourself. It also puts you at the risk of getting caught up in all the unreason that goes with our profession.

My point today is not that medicine is impossibly dangerous, or that you're particularly vulnerable. It is simply that in order to deal with normal slings and arrows, doctors tend to use certain defense mechanisms more than others, and understanding them can help you pay attention to getting care for yourselves in order to care for others. Physician, cherish thyself.

RECOMMENDED READING

Bittker, Thomas E., 1979, "Why Can't We Heed A Colleague's Cry For Help?" *Medical Economics*, Vol. 56, No. 16, pp. 73–78.

Carlson, Gabrielle, A., and Miller, Diana C., 1981, "Suicide, Affective Disorder, and Women Physicians," *American Journal of Psychiatry*, Vol. 138, No. 10, pp. 1330–1334.

Jefferson, Linda V., and Ensor, Barbara E., 1982, "Help for the Helper: Confronting a Chemically-Impaired Colleague," *American Journal of Nursing*, April Issue, pp. 574–577.

Levine, Carol, 1983, "Dealing With Impaired Physicians," *Medica*, Winter, 1983, pp. 23, 24, 34.

Lipp, Martin R., 1980, *The Bitter Pill*, Harper & Row, New York, 204 pp.

Pasnau, Robert O., and Russell, Andrew T., 1975, "Psychiatric Resident Suicide: An Analysis of Five Cases," *American Journal of Psychiatry*, Vol. 132, No. 4, pp. 402–405.

Pepitone-Arreola-Rockwell, Fran, Rockwell, Don, and Core, Nolan, 1981, "Fifty-Two Medical Student Suicides," *American Journal of Psychiatry*, Vol. 138, No. 2, pp. 198–201.

Rosenberg, Charlotte L., 1979, "Doctor Rehabilitation: It *Is* Working," *Medical Economics*, Vol. 56, No. 25, pp. 114–122.

Scheiber, Stephen C., and Doyle, Brian B., 1983, *The Impaired Physician*, Plenum Medical Book Co., New York, 211 pp.

Thomas, Caroline Bedell, 1976, "What Becomes of Medical Students: The Dark Side," *The Johns Hopkins Medical Journal*, Vol. 138, No. 5, May Issue, pp. 186–195.

Vaillant, George E., Sobowaler, Nancy Corbin, and McArthur, Charles, 1972, "Some Psychologic Vulnerabilities of Physicians," *The New England Journal of Medicine*, Vol. 287, No. 8, pp. 372–375.

5

Compleat Physicians: Balancing Hands, Head, and Heart

If physician impairement is to be understood, it's opposite must also be recognized. "Compleat Physicians," with the old English spelling for emphasis, is the name we give physicians who, in contrast to their impaired colleagues, maintain a healthy balance between work and other life aspects. They are well-balanced and healthy.

"The longer I live," observed Oliver Wendell Holmes, "the more I am satisfied of two things: first, that the truest lives are those that are cut rose-diamond fashion, with many faces answering to the many-planed aspects of the world about them; secondly, that society is always trying in some way or other to grind us down to a single flat surface. It is hard work to resist this grinding down action."

Compleat physicians have resisted this grinding down process by balancing their careers with other life activities. They have successfully avoided being swept along by social forces that promote excessive career involvement at the expense of personal and familial well-being. By thoughtfully setting personal goals in a variety of life domains, these physicians have become well-rounded. In addition to career involvements, their time and energy has been devoted to activities that promote physical and emotional fitness, spiritual and cultural sensitivity, and social and familial vitality. Such doctors are at ease in social settings where medicine is not the primary topic of conversation.

"Impaired doctors" and "compleat physicians" are, of course, ideal types. In reality, few physicians actually fit either of these extreme descriptions; most vary in degrees on a continuum between these opposites. But all are gradually moving toward one type or the other. Compleatness or impairment is a developmental process, not an event; professional careers are dynamic, not static.

A model of compleat professional development is represented by three overlapping circles, each symbolizing an interdependent area of personal competence vital to physician effectiveness. The first circle represents mental discipline, the cognitive know-how for accurate diagnosis and appropriate intervention; the second symbolizes the manual skills necessary to carrying out clinical tests and procedures; and the third symbolizes the affective aspects of patient care, the ability to develop rapport and deal compassionately with patients. Because all of these areas of professional competence are interdependent—the intellect (head), clinical skills (hands), and patient–physician affect (heart)—impaired performance results when one or more is underdeveloped. Compleat professionals are disciplined in all three.

Because the system of medical training typically emphasizes only two of these domains—the head and the hands—it is easy to neglect one's own emotional development. Though knowledgeable and technically competent, the emerging physician's lifestyle and personality can become unbalanced.

When devoting excessive amounts of time and energy to career activities, "outside" involvements become minimal. By gradually severing ties with family members and neglecting restorative activities that offer rest and diversion, emotional resilience is diminished. When this occurs, the technical quality of work suffers, as do relationships with patients and others. These unrewarding encounters contribute to greater frustration, thus bringing about a vicious cycle.

In the pursuit of excellence, in constantly attempting to impress critical colleagues, and thereby feel good about oneself, a physician's lifestyle can become skewed, imbalanced. When one is overworked and preoccupied with career concerns, physical and emotional exhaustion are likely. This condition is exacerbated when, in order to project a proper image, personal feelings of doubt, uncertainty, fear, and personal inadequacy are chronically suppressed.

How much more simple and effective to avoid these debilitating processes by maintaining a more balanced approach. But, as Oliver Wendell Holmes has pointed out, "It is not easy nor come naturally to live a well-balanced life. Two obstacles usually stand in the way. First is our own failure to thoughtfully determine what is of greatest value and set goals—determine what we want out of life and how much effort each should receive. The second is the social pressure that favors one or more of these values to the exclusion of the others."

"Whenever men attempt," Bernard Baruch observed, "They seem driven to overdo." This potential for extremes and excesses is present, of course, in all human endeavors. Significant accomplishment requires considerable time and effort, but balance, production, and reflective planning are needed to rise to full potential. Compleat physicians pause often enough, long enough, to appraise what is of greatest value, and then budget their time and energies to ensure viable growth in all important areas. That is, the career of a compleat physician, though important, does not dominate other vital aspects of living. Work activities are kept within the healthy limits of moderation, a virtue which has been called "the silk string through the pearl chain of all virtues." In maintaining a balance, these physicians avoid becoming narrow, lopsided personalities and, as such, become more, not less, effective in their careers.

Like the columns of a businessperson's financial ledger, success cannot be measured by high attainment on only one column, especially when achieved at the expense of the other columns. It must be measured horizontally—by assessing all important columns. Similarly, compleat physicians regard success horizontally, considering all dimensions of their lives, not just careers. Little admired are their medical colleagues who, though they have attained honorific professional status, have done so at the expense of their personal and familial well-being. If one is to be judged truly successful—compleat—all of life's important dimensions must be kept in balanced proportion.

Dealing sensitively with others' feelings, cannot, of course, be achieved if, in the pursuit of career attainment, one's own emotional well-being has been neglected. A personal life devoid of emotional sensitivity is not likely to be one that contains the range and depth of experiences necessary for a humanistic clinical practice or for a personal life characterized by growth and fulfillment. The emotionally uneducated, those who have developed only the "head" and "hands" but neglected the "heart," will, as Donald Arnstein has said, "live most of their emotional lives as children, taking seriously what deserves a smile, laughing at what deserves respect, and floating on the surface of experience, the depth of which is hidden to them."

How can one maintain emotional well-being when besieged with work demands? For most physicians, the simplest and most profound way is to establish and cultivate a viable long-term relationship with a caring, emotionally expressive spouse. The lack of such a companion is an interpersonal deficit that makes one vulnerable to stress.

At work, one is judged primarily on the basis of achievement. At home, one is valued intrinsically. That is, mates and other family members place more emphasis upon *who you are* than *what you can do*. A durable relationship with an accepting, emotionally expressive mate provides a reprieve, a regular retreat from competitive, demanding situations at work where one is constantly "on stage," performing before a critical audience. Such companions rejoice in each other's successes and stand by one another in defeat, failure, and loss. When one has such a viable companionship, emotional regression is unlikely.

Unlike "roadside romances" that quickly flourish and wither like flowers along the roadside, such relationships do not develop quickly and are not maintained successfully without effort. Like careers and cultivated gardens, they must be carefully planned and nurtured regularly; when neglected, they can become unsightly.

If one sacrifices family and balanced living for career attainment, dreaming of a "golden day" ahead, one may miss it all; for success, like happiness, is a journey, not an outcome.

But won't an outlay of time and energy for family place yet another burden on an already demanding schedule? After all, there are only so many hours in a day. It is our view that, by taking time away from work to stay physically and emotionally fit, one may accomplish more, not less. A rested, emotionally restored physician, one who understands his or her own feelings and those of family members, will, in all likelihood, be more—not less—energetic, effective, and compassionate at work.

In Maslow's "hierarchy of human needs," the need for love and belonging immediately follows that of food and shelter. Of the various mechanisms society has established to meet this need, marriage and family are the most universal and can be, with planning and effort, the most fulfilling. Campbell (1981, p. 73) has noted that it is hard to imagine an individual who is immersed in an unhappy marriage living a pleasant and satisfying life. By the same token, it is difficult to imagine a physician engaged in a happy, emotionally expressive marriage who is unproductive and unful- filled either at home *or* at work.

What about women physicians? Do these generalizations apply to them? If women are more emotionally expressive, are they more likely to become compleat physicians?

In the 1970s the women's movement began to focus on the male-dominated medical profession, pointing out that it was offering insensitive, inadequate care especially to women. Some women argued that only female physicians could solve this problem, because women tend to be more sensitive and nurturing, more caring. Eventually, the doors to medical school began to open to women, and gradually increasing numbers have been admitted.

Once admitted, a variety of problems have confronted women, such as gaining respect from male colleagues and the trust and confidence of patients. From history most people expect women to be nurses, not doctors. Dealing with such stereotypes has been a daily burden to many women. "Some patients don't believe me when I introduce myself as doctor," one lamented. "They hear me say I'm Doctor Jones, but they think I really *meant* to say I'm a nurse."

In order for a woman to function as a physician, she must reject the sex-linked stereotype of feminine passivity, dependence, and submission. She must also convince her male colleagues *and* her patients that she is at least as good as a male doctor. In doing this tightrope act, she risks being perceived as "strident." For the same behavior for which a man would be regarded as "assertive," a woman might be labeled as "bitchy."

Some studies have shown physician impairment to be higher for women than men. If accurate, does this mean that women, traditionally regarded as the "weaker sex," just can't handle the stresses of the medical profession? Or does it mean their stress is greater and/or their support system weaker? We think it is clearly the latter. For one thing, a woman doctor rarely has a "wife" at home to provide nurturing support and household relief—taking care of household chores, raising the children, cooking, and being readily accessible to provide relief for whatever problems arise. Men are taught instrumental, work-, or task-oriented behaviors based on the ability to compete, be strong, dominant, and independent. Compared to women, men are less often taught to be nurturant and supportive of their spouses, or to help with household chores.

The woman doctor, then, may face not only everyday problems with her male colleagues and with her patients, but also with her husband. Without realizing it, he may expect her, though a busy physician, to be a traditional wife as well. And if they have children, you can bet that she feels pressure to be a traditional mother; in all likelihood, she expects it of herself. Many career women, not just physicians, labor under the notion that they must, to be considered worthy human beings, be experts not only in their careers but in all of the traditional "women's work" areas. In short, they must be Superwoman, and they judge themselves to be failures if they do not excel at all of these jobs. Society (and their mothers-in-law) expect them to be superb housekeepers, cooks, mothers, Scout leaders, etc., and other doctors expect them to be superb physicians and resent any requests for "special favors"—such as time off for child-related problems. After all, *they* don't allow *their* personal and family problems to interfere with *their* work. Of course not—their wives handle those problems. Small wonder, then, that some women who try to be all of these things—doctor, supportive wife, mother, housekeeper, laundress, cook, and so on—collapse emotionally under the weight, especially if their mates are demanding critics rather than emotionally supportive companions.

These issues are addressed in the first selection, "Observations on Women in Medicine," by Donna K. Whitney, our esteemed UCLA colleague.

In an address to prospective women physicians, Whitney urges resistance to the subtle pressures that "inexorably leaches out" from young professionals much that is soft, tender, humble, and creative to be replaced by an unnatural cockiness and bruskness. She cautions that if doctors don't want to become "hardened" they had better not change their personalities just for the years of medical school and residency, because it isn't so easy to change back into a caring human being once in practice. "The habits we cultivate during our training become our habits for the years to come," she explains. Her advice to women is that they be the best doctors *and* the best women they can.

The second selection, "Teaching Physical Diagnosis—Emotions and Privileges," by Rich Davis, underscores the need for emotional sensitivity in clinical practice. Typically, he says, courses and textbooks tend to ignore the psychological processes and emotions that are stirred within patients during a physical examination— feelings bordering on helplessness when submitting to nakedness, cold instruments, and intimate exposures previously kept to one's own discretion. Because of the Herculean work load imposed on young doctors, Davis emphasizes, it is easy to become calloused to patient examinations, "to treat it as routine, as an academic fact-finding tour, and to forget the fears invariably hidden behind the frequent patient smiles." He urges medical educators to keep the human dimension in mind, in order to produce the kind of compassionate and considerate clinicians we call compleat physicians. "Remember doc," one patient remarked, "there's a person in here!"

The stages that medical trainees evolve through in dealing with their feelings is explored in the next article entitled, "Socialization for Death: The Physician's Role." Coombs and Powers address the question of how one maintains a professional demeanor, keeping one's feelings under control, without becoming hardened and desensitized to patients' feelings and suggest that physicians progress through predictable stages in dealing with patient-related emotions. The first stage is one of idealism in which medical trainees react emotionally much as laymen. In the second stage, medical students become desensitized to "death symbols"—blood, bones, corpses, etc. During the third stage, prospective doctors disassociate themselves not only from the death symbols, but also from the emotions that surround suffering and death. Then, as an antithesis to the first three stages, some but not all physicians begin to question their "dehumanized" perspectives (stage 4) and finally come to grips with their own feelings (stage 5).

Although the system of medical education inevitably takes trainees through the first three stages, those who advance to stage 5, compleat physicians, typically do so with little or no institutional encouragement. How much better if, at each stage, fledgling physicians were encouraged to explore the affective component (heart) at the same time they were experiencing their academic and clinical training (head and hands)—i.e., to experience stages 4 and 5 concomitantly with the first three. Then trainees would leave the training institutions as compleat young physicians well disciplined in head, hands, *and* heart.

The final articles, both medical school commencement addresses, clearly illustrate the possibility of achieving stages 4 and 5 during medical school. Each author, a graduating fourth-year student, is critical of those aspects of the training system which promote imbalanced living and emotional constriction.

Selected by his classmates at the University of California, San Francisco, to give the senior class graduation address, Scott May encouraged physicians to maintain a balance between "male principles" (e.g., competition, aggression, logic, intellect) and "female principles" (e.g., receptivity, creativity, sensitivity, and nurturance). Medical practice, he says, is not just a succession of traumatic emergencies, but "human stories involving souls and feelings." Nurturance, tenderness, and soulfulness—the qualities patients want in their physicians—get crowded out in medical school by perfection, evaluation, and demand for performance. A technological rather than a humanistic emphasis too often alienates physicians from their patients. Professional distance, he says, can become interpersonal coldness and arrogance.

At a similar event across the country, Mark Wenneker, a graduating senior at Harvard Medical School, also encouraged his classmates to strive for balance rather than total career commitment. Does becoming "a shaker and a mover" in medicine, a future leader, he asks, require one to forsake all else, to devote one's life to medicine? Must one prefer the care of patients to eating, sleeping, and other recreational activities? No, he answers, and titles his address, "Rebelling Against Big Brother." One can become a leader in medicine, he asserts and still not lose sight of other priorities. At the very least, he projects, "we will be competent physicians with meaningful lives."

REFERENCE

Campbell, Angus, 1981, *The Sense of Well-Being in America*, New York, McGraw-Hill.

Observations on Women in Medicine

Donna K. Whitney

In considering issues related to women in medicine, frequently we hear discussion of discrimination regarding medical school admissions, residency selections, faculty appointments, and academic advancement. We hear also about the effect of gender upon choice of specialty, referral patterns, and income. I will say at the outset that I have no knowledge of the statistics on these topics, little desire to learn them, and no intention of discussing them. My concern is with the people who study and practice medicine. How do they respond to the challenges of their profession, how do they change and grow? What becomes of their values, their ethics, their personalities, their beliefs? With regard to these issues, I am concerned equally with male physicians and females, even though in some ways the two genders probably experience these issues differently.

By now you may have heard it said that medical education and training are as much a process of being socialized as of being instructed. I would agree that there are certain normative beliefs and mores which are subtly but firmly urged upon us during the progressive rites of initiation into the profession, and I would contend that these values and mores tend toward the masculine rather than the feminine. We learn to speak with power rather than with authority, to give commands rather than to speak, to demand rather than suggest, to cure rather than to heal. These values and nuances of personal style can advance so insidiously as to go unnoticed until they are well established in the medical initiate. I personally have observed the gradual but inexorable leaching out of much that is soft, tender, humble, and creative from young physicians, to be replaced by an unnatural cockiness and brusqueness. I have observed this in myself, and have sometimes been surprised to hear myself speak with a voice that is not my own.

The pressures may be subtle, but they are strong. The physician or student who lingers at the bedside and is late for rounds faces a certain disapproval. The doctor who rules out bodily injury and then goes on further to initiate personal counseling for a rape victim may appear unproductive in a busy emergency room. There are choices at every turn—between efficiency and humanity, patient care and rounds, clinical dedication and academic excellence. But the crux of the matter is this, that there is always a choice, and only I can choose for myself. Others can exert pressures, but make no mistake, my choices are mine alone, and so are the consequences.

When I say mine *alone*, or yours alone, I would emphasize *alone*. Much of in-hospital medicine is practiced in the abundant and often unwanted company of others. I certainly dislike struggling to hear myself think in the cacophony of a dozen conversations and half a dozen beepers going all at once. But in spite of the flocking and herding patterns of rounds and conferences, much of our career consists of time spent alone. Alone at night on call, alone with a suffering patient, alone with a peculiar chest X-ray or smudged gram stain, alone with a questioning relative, alone with the imperative to do something in the face of uncertainty—the most significant part of our professional lives is spent alone. It is in this solitary silence that I confront and know and create myself again and again. I say create because I believe we determine who we become by what we choose and what we do.

This brings me to another major issue in the professional development of physicians of both sexes. As a medical student, I often heard it said that the rigors of clerkship, internship, and residency demanded a certain hardened attitude and sacrificing of human niceties, but that once in practice—presumably in a plush office in Beverly Hills or its equivalent—we could relax again in the luxuriant lap of income and autonomy to become the compassionate, honest selves we started out to be and always intended to be. This simply isn't so. What we do determines what we become, and the habits we cultivate during our training become our habits for the years to come. The only way to become compassionate is to practice compassion; the only way to become honest is to practice honesty; the only way to become a thief is to commit theft.

These are the issues which are vital to me, and they transcend gender distinctions and are not unique to medicine. I care as much about how my male colleagues confront them as I do about how other women confront them. So why, then, did I choose to talk about these things in a conversation about women in medicine?

First of all, the challenges of personal and professional growth and ethics are greatly heightened in medicine in a compelling way. I am sure that my own internship brought me face to face with moral and personal issues which I would otherwise not have taken on until later in life. Secondly, the challenges of personal and professional integrity in medicine impact upon women differently from men, and raise the opportunity for inquiry into the actualization of our feminine selves in the superficially masculine world of medicine.

On one occasion, I heard Doctor Ed Johnson, the Associate Dean of Students at Southwestern Medical School, speak before a gathering similar to this one in Dallas, Texas. Dr. Johnson is a more practical and patient person than I am, and he began with some discouraging numbers about women in academic medicine. Then he went on to discuss the immense sacrifices women had to make in order to become successful academic physicians in positions of power. Their marriages suffered; they felt inadequate as mothers, or maybe never became mothers at all; their family and personal lives became sterile; some acknowledged that in a fundamental human way, they felt diminished. Somehow it all seemed so unfair. But then, Dr. Johnson went on to examine the life-choices of male academics in prestigious positions. Their marriages, their relationships with their children, their effectiveness and fulfillment outside the realm of academic medicine also suffered. We can easily look around us and find men for whom these sad consequences apply. We women have developed an unbecoming habit of complaining about these choices of ours, and about the consequences, and we have even developed a narrowness of vision which lets us believe these choices are faced only by women. What is different for women is not the sets of choices with which we are confronted, but our awareness of the choosing and our feelings about the consequences. Awareness and feeling are nothing to complain about. They are, as a pair, a source of tremendous power with which we can cultivate our integrity, effectiveness and fulfillment, both professionally and personally.

It is not because we are women, but because we are human that we must do so much choosing. As women, however, we may bring to our decisions not only a special awareness and feeling, but also our own values. Of course, there is enormous individual variation in personal values, and generalizations about the two sexes can be made tentatively at best. Nonetheless, I think that women more than men will tend to value service to others above individual fortune, and family above career. If this proves to be so when somebody gets around to looking at the statistics, I for one will be neither resentful nor ashamed. Similarly, if it turns out that female doctors take more thorough histories, perform more meticulous physical examinations, touch their patients more, and simply enjoy their work more—and my own casual observation would suggest that it is so—I would find no cause in this either for shame.

If we are to find some fulfillment as women doctors, we must shrink neither from being doctors nor from being women. There really is, I believe, a motive to avoid success in women, as popularized in the doctoral thesis of Matina Horner. We need to be aware of this in ourselves, as it interferes with our becoming the doctors we want to be. We can actualize ourselves as women in medicine not by straining to match our numbers, ideas, words, voices, values, and choices with men, but by allowing our choices to flow from our authentic, aware, feeling, valuing feminine selves, and letting the numbers fall as they may.

Teaching Physical Diagnosis— Emotions and Privileges

Rich Davis

Although the primary purpose of any text or course in physical diagnosis is to enlighten the learner about successful methods of physical diagnosis, there should be an important, if somewhat secondary, purpose. That is to alert and educate the learner about the psychological process occurring and the emotions being stirred during a physical examination. The great majority of both texts and courses tend to ignore the emotional dimension engendered by one human physically and verbally probing another. Yet physician–patient interaction is rarely more delicately experienced, at least by the patient, than during a physical examination.

All that a physician need do to refresh the intense personal significance of such an experience is to submit to it by a fellow physician. However sophisticated and educated he or she may be, there is a feeling, at times bordering on helplessness, as one submits to nakedness, cold instruments, and casual, if professional, disinterest in those exposures we have so preciously kept to our own discretion. A personal physical examination for the physician is an abrupt reminder for him of what every person experiences during any physical examination.

I still recall a woman (of what some call the world's oldest profession) fearfully and angrily clasping her clothes to her bare front (anterior) as I foolishly walked into the examining room without first knocking. "Get your ass (posterior) out of here until I'm dressed!" she shouted. And I did. She later reminded me that although this may have been my tenth examination that day, it was her first in a year. I have never forgotten her reminder that each patient's examination is unique, important, and highly personal (regardless of profession). Although one should not become preoccupied with patients' fears and anxieties, becoming so occupied with physical findings and the science of medicine that such emotions are ignored represents failure to practice the art of medicine.

The novice physician has such a huge task of learning that it is easy for the most sensitive and compassionate to become too accustomed to patient examination, to treat it as routine, as an academic fact-finding tour, and to forget the fears invariably hidden behind the frequent patient smiles. It is similarly easy for us to take for granted the rare privilege extended to us by society and the individual patient, when they permit us, even encourage us, to examine and question that which, if another unlicensed person were to do, would probably lead to arrest, jail, and conviction for assault and battery.

These privileges are truly remarkable, nearly global, and risked with few human beings in this world.

With the patient's permission, we are given the legal and moral right to take a piece of sharp steel and jab into another's flesh, to slice open the belly of a fellow human being and sew it back up after examining the bowels, or after removing vital organs, to handle the most private parts of another human body, and to ask the most intimate questions. Secrets shared with us may not be shared within the most private councils of the patient's family. We are permitted to ask a relative stranger of either sex to disrobe, to assume the most awkward and humiliating of positions, to accept the introduction of foreign objects into any orifice, often to tolerate considerable discomfort or even pain, and yet they are expected to express no resistance, only cooperation.

In short, with proper credentials and the permission of an individual, we are permitted to do things that no one else may do.

Unavoidably, these rare privileges are accompanied over the years by equally awesome responsibilities to remain sensitive and considerate of the patient's feelings, both emotional and physical, to adequately inform the patient of the reasons and purposes for such examinations and treatments, and to understand ahead of time that however well motivated our actions are, they may at times be misunderstood by frightened or angry people.

This combination of unique privileges and responsibilities demands not only that one develop skill in physically examining a patient, but that one develop his or her own personality, character, and stability to the point where all requests of the patient are consistently addressed for the patient's benefit, and not as overt or disguised means of rewarding the physician's need for approval or advantage.

Should the physician come to view himself other than as a servant to the sick, one who waits upon and serves others, he or she will distort that role. A physician certainly is not subservient to the patient, but his activities should only enhance his self-esteem in parallel with his humility. This nearly sacred trust that the public has placed in the physician is there for one reason only—to assist the human being who is ill and disadvantaged in understanding what is wrong, and to take appropriate measures to correct it. Dr. Karl Menninger expressed this well.

> It might be summed up as one (attitude) of respect for the dignity of the individual human being and of reverence for the mystery of pain, of impaired life and growth. With this, too, goes respect for the responsibility and authority of the role of the physician—a self-respect, and the respect for one's associates and their predecessors, for the accumulation of medical science, and for the quality and the nature of human beings that leads them to turn in trust to some of their equally fallible fellow creatures and place their fate in our hands. Such respect dictates a pervasive humility and an earnest dedication to a task approaching a function of divinity.[1]

Therefore, medical educators should encourage students to keep the human dimension in mind while learning the facts and skills necessary to diagnose disease adequately and to treat compassionately our fellow humans. Such a dimension formally interwoven throughout a classical text in physical diagnosis, or in a course in physical diagnosis, or in our own daily practice, is one compatible with the best in medical practice, where the art and the science of medicine are so entwined as to produce a compassionate medical scientist, the kind of considerate and well-trained human being we all hope it is our privilege to know when we are the patient who is being examined.

NOTE

1. Menninger, K., 1952, *A Manual for Psychiatric Case Study*, New York, Grune & Stratton.

Socialization for Death:
The Physician's Role

Robert H. Coombs and Pauline S. Powers

In days gone by, death was a family experience. In the hamlets and villages of rural America, people usually died at home attended by family members and friends of long acquaintance. At the moment of death, these intimate associates were often present, providing comforting care, exchanging meaningful words, and then observing the termination of breathing and the total relaxation of the body.[1]

In striking contrast, death in the contemporary urban setting now occurs primarily in hospitals and other medical facilities. Only rarely are family members or friends present during the final moments of life. Instead, the dying are attended by medical and paramedical specialists, each highly trained to perform technical services in combating disease and death. Presiding over this staff of technical experts is the attending physician. He is the commander-in-chief, the one authoritative figure recognized by others as inevitably concerned with dying and death. Not only does he orchestrate the clinical efforts of staff, but he is also required by his presiding role to decide when the patient is dead (an increasingly complex decision), to sign the death certificate, and then to confront the family with the news.

It is no easy matter to learn this difficult role successfully, for potentially conflicting demands are often placed upon the physician.[2] He is not only expected to be expert in applying highly specialized technical skills, but he also must treat the patient—and his family—with gentleness and sympathy. His main job is to cure if possible, but he must also relieve and comfort. All of medicine's scientific advances have not eliminated the patient's need for warm sensitivity and understanding concern.

But the doctor cannot take death and dying too personally: he is expected to retain composure, no matter how dramatic or tragic the death scene might be. Rationality and clearness of judgment in moments of grave peril must characterize his every action. The physician who loses coolness and presence of mind also loses the confidence of patients and staff. Clearly, a doctor sobbing over a favorite patient is no doctor at all.

STUDYING THE SOCIALIZATION OF PHYSICIANS

To understand how physicians-in-training master the complexities of the clinical role pertaining to death and dying, we have utilized extensive data derived from longitudinal interviews and participant observation. The primary source of information comes from a panel analysis of an entire class of medical students who entered medical school in the fall of 1967 and exited in June 1971 with the M.D. degree. During each year of training, members of the class were interviewed about their changing attitudes toward death and dying.[3] Two hundred and twenty-nine tape-recorded interviews, of a possible 239, were obtained, all but two of which were personally conducted by the senior author. These interviews were transcribed, coded, and tabulated.

Enriching these longitudinal data are field notes derived from participant observation at the medical school and teaching hospital. By accompanying students as they went about their activities, additional insights were generated to supplement the interview information. These observations were in turn checked against the observations of the second author, who only recently had personally experienced the status passage through successive stages of medical training—medical school, internship, and residency. The second author also conducted tape-recorded interviews with 13 of her medical colleagues.[4] These intensive interviews not only provided insights concerning socialization experiences during the latter stages of training (that is, internship and residency), but also gave retrospective views of how medical training affects later clinical practice.

DEVELOPMENTAL STAGES IN DEALING WITH DEATH

In the medical school and teaching hospital, medical aspirants learn the physician's role. Here recruits are processed through a series of challenging experiences which, if encountered successfully, transform them from laymen into effective physicians. Described in sociological terms, the medical center is a formal socializing system whose function it is to prepare participants for the physician's role—a role which requires considerable expertise in dealing with death and dying.[5]

Our thesis is that, in learning to deal with this sensitive subject, medical practitioners evolve through fairly predictable developmental stages. While these stages are not inevitable, we suggest that they are representative of the developmental changes which typically occur as laymen change into seasoned clinical practitioners.

Stage I: Idealizing the Doctor's Role

Upon beginning medical training, students have essentially the same attitudes and feelings about death as the general public. Having had little personal experience with death and dying, students are no more enlightened than others. Like laymen, they regard the doctor as a bulwark against death and suffering. In their minds, death is the antithesis of good medical practice. "That's my business," a freshman said, "to make sure death doesn't occur."

Emotionally, too, beginning students differ little from laymen in the way they respond to death. They have not escaped the fears and phobias which beset others. Obviously, death can be a shocking experience, and students are not immune to the normal emotional reactions which occur on such occasions. To deal routinely with dying people, as they must learn to do, requires coping skills which they have not yet developed.[6]

At this pre-professional stage, personal identification with dying patients is strong, especially if the latter are young and likable, and students are apt to find themselves participating imaginatively in the suffering involved. They have not yet evolved from the layman's attitude toward suffering and death. In time, however, they will begin to acquire the detachment and equanimity of the veteran doctor, which many of them realize. Nonetheless, this transition can be quite painful. Intellectual understanding is one thing, but managing feelings is quite another.

Initially, students find the coolness of the case-hardened clinician offensive. In their idealistic view, the physician, like the proverbial country doctor, should be warm and compassionate. So it is disillusioning to witness the detachment which is typically exhibited in the hospital setting. For example, when one freshman was given an opportunity to accompany upper-classmen on ward rounds, he was appalled by the "unfeeling way" the attending physician talked to the group about a terminally ill patient. "I'd sure hate to have the family hear him talk like that," he said. "I suppose the doctor has to be uncompassionate at times, but I wasn't ready for it. He wasn't disrespectful, but he just didn't show any emotion."

Similarly, a sophomore was shocked at the detached attitude of the staff about the death of his first patient. Unaware of her death, he had tried to locate her in the hospital room and was told matter of factly, "She's in the morgue." "This really bothered me," he confessed. "I went to her autopsy and it made me think pretty deeply for awhile."

Another student was appalled by the scientific interest displayed by the clinical staff who attended his first patient, a baby who was unsuccessfully operated on for a congenital cardiac anomaly: "The surgeon was sorry, I guess, but it was kind of a scientific study to him; things like this evidently happen every week or two." Later, during the autopsy, this student was stunned when the pediatric cardiologist was "real excited when the autopsy findings compared well with his own diagnosis."

Upsetting as these experiences are, most students realize, at least on an intellectual level, that such detachment does not necessarily indicate a lack of concern, and that, in fact, a doctor's failure to become emotionally involved may be in the best interests of the patient. Later on, in fact, these same students may find themselves reacting to death much like their mentors, but at this initial stage they typically respond as do laymen.

Stage II: Desensitizing Death Symbols

From the beginning of medical training, students are conditioned in the art of remaining emotionally aloof in the face of human tragedy. In medical practice, death is omnipresent, and the prospective doctor must be desensitized to its symbols—blood, bones, corpses, and stench—symbols which are disturbing to most people.[7] Although many students have had some desensitizing experiences in their pre-med courses which require them to dissect and sometimes even kill living things, medical school experiences can be shocking.

Almost the moment students arrive in medical school, they are escorted into the anatomy laboratory and introduced to a cadaver, a dead body which they are expected to cut into and dissect in careful detail. Not surprisingly, most students initially feel shock and revulsion upon seeing a room full of dead bodies lying lifeless and gray on steel tables. Few, if any, can carry off such a confrontation with complete sang-froid. Rather, the initial reaction is typically masked by a sense of nausea triggered by the heavy smell of formaldehyde, a sense of recoil upon finding the corpse so cold and rigid to first touch, and a feeling of depression, a loss of appetite, and an inability to concentrate after the first encounter.

But no matter how great the initial shock, it apparently wears off rapidly since most students claim to adjust quickly. Only three of our cohort indicated that more than a week was required to reestablish their emotional equilibrium. Of the latter, one experienced severe anxiety, another was not able to touch the cadaver until he had put on rubber gloves, and the third sought medical treatment for an allergic reaction.

It is not long, however, until students become so desensitized that they can eat their lunches around the corpse. It is important to realize, though, that the ability to undergo such experiences without betraying disgust or squeamishness is a valued characteristic among prospective doctors. This desire to portray nonchalance, to remain "cool," no doubt causes students to exaggerate the ease with which discomforting experiences are met and, in turn, to suppress openness about personal anxieties. The fact that students frequently have bad dreams about the cadaver experience suggests that they do have repressed anxieties.[8]

To manage these anxieties and thereby make the experience more tolerable, students utilize a number of coping mechanisms. One is humor, a ready tension release.[9] Despite faculty efforts to discourage pranks and horseplay, amusing stories about the cadaver circulate among students. They jokingly give amusing names to the lifeless forms, or contrive the body in such a way as to get a laugh—for example, arranging an erect penis on a female student's cadaver. Such antics function as a tension release and also help students forget the morose aspects of the experience.

The challenge to the neophyte doctor is, of course, to keep his personal sensitivities intact while dissecting a human body. Humanistically inclined students, those most prone to worrying about the moral justifications of carving into a cadaver, find relief in the knowledge that patients have willingly donated their own bodies to be used in training medical students.

Inner relief is most typically derived, though, by losing oneself in the details of the work. The pressure to learn myriad body parts in a limited time reinforces the tendency among students to occupy themselves with the finite details of the dissection process and in memorizing the scientific names of bones, muscles, nerves, and other body parts. In so doing, dissection becomes a mechanistic exercise rather than a humanistic experience. This absorption in work clearly acts, to use Lief and Fox's term (1963), as a "psychic non-irritant."

Further desensitization occurs in the second year when students are introduced to pathology and experience their first autopsy. One might suppose this experience to be little different from the cadaver experience. But an autopsy brings students much closer to the subjective or personal aspects of death because the body, only a few hours earlier, was living![10] So it is much easier to identify with the deceased. This personal involvement is enhanced by the fact that, as compared with a cadaver, the body is left heavily draped and appears much more lifelike. Moreover, unlike the cadaver experience, students have knowledge of the patient's identity and medical history through reading the patient's chart and listening to the doctor's report about the fatal illness.

In order to maintain equanimity and protect themselves from the discomfort of such a stressful experience, students, like their mentors, adopt a detached scientific attitude. That is, emotionality is avoided or suppressed by focusing on the technical aspects of their work. Losing oneself in the pathological details of an autopsy helps prospective doctors maintain an "objective professional response." Clearly, thinking about diseased tissue is less emotionally involving than pondering about the patient as a person.

Required basic-science courses in the freshman and sophomore years provide the scientific terminology and knowledge necessary for dealing with illness on an intellectual rather than an emotional basis. Through constant exposure to scientific aspects of disease, these courses desensitize students to disease processes, the precursors of death. Reflecting on such a course, a physician said, "It's just hours and hours of looking at slides of people who have various illnesses at progressive stages. It's like looking at war scenes again and again until after a while it doesn't have the same emotional content."

At this stage, then, the prospective doctor is prepared, psychologically, to deal with the aversive symbols of death without displaying emotionality (fear, revulsion, and so forth). By becoming desensitized to blood, bones, and other symbols of death which normally elicit uncomfortable feelings, he comes closer to the expected professional response—a calm, objective rationality and a full control of emotion. This conditioning prepares him for the face-to-face encounters he will have with living patients.

Stage III: Objectifying and Combating Death

When the training scene shifts from the lecture room and laboratory to the hospital, students are exposed to some of life's most poignant dramas. Everywhere present are the companions of death—pain, suffering, fear, and despair. Here students learn to distance themselves emotionally from the living as well as the dead.

Early experiences with dying patients make clear the necessity of detaching oneself from the emotional trauma of death. "It's really hard the first two or three times a patient dies," a senior student explained; "so you learn to develop a protective shield to reduce the emotional impact." Consider, for example, the strain that this stressful experience might have on a fledgling doctor:

> My first patient was a little boy suffering from incurable leukemia. He was all right when he left the hospital, but in about two weeks he came into the emergency room in shock and died three hours later. When I was in the room with him, the attending physician asked, "Who had this patient before?" When I told him I had, he sent me to look after the mother who was crying in the next room. While the doctor worked on the little 5-year-old, I tried to talk to the mother. I really felt terribly inadequate; there wasn't a whole lot I could say to make her feel better. Then we went into the room where they were treating the boy. He was screaming and crying and then stopped breathing. The mother collapsed and somebody caught her. That experience really got to me!

Such happenings make clear to students the necessity of developing coping mechanisms which will allow them to do their work without getting "all wrapped up" in the patients' lives. The main depersonalizing technique, modeled effectively by the clinical faculty, is to objectify death, or, conversely, deny the subjective features. In other words, the clinician learns to view dying patients not as people with feelings, but as medical entities, specimens, or objects of scientific interest. By adopting a scientific frame of mind, utilized so effectively in their previous work with dead bodies, clinicians can effectively avoid the uncomfortable inner feelings which occur when they are exposed to dying patients. In this way, as a fourth-year student points out, "Death can be as neutral as reading the obituary section of the newspaper."[11]

The dynamics by which clinicians dissociate themselves involve an intellectual dissection of the patient into parts and then concentrating on and treating only the pathological part rather than the "whole person." "This is the old scientific fragmentalization method," an experienced physician explained. "You just bust up the human organism into pieces and deal only with the pieces. Then you don't have to see the whole picture." It is this orientation which expresses itself in such comments as "the liver in room 724" or "an interesting case of leukemia."

Obviously there is much less discomfort for a physician in the "expiration" of a "case" than in the death of a patient. Similarly, the "emotional horror" of dealing with a 9-year-old boy dying from a head injury is less stressful, as one physician acknowledged, when concentrating on the anatomy and physiological processes. "That's the model that was driven into me," he recalled.

This is not to say, however, that doctors take lightly their clinical responsibilities. On the contrary, heavy demands are routinely made upon medical trainees to be exhaustively thorough in trying to keep people alive and well. Before a person dies there is usually a "mad scramble," as one put it, to get everything possible done to save him. When a patient stops breathing or his heart stops beating, an emergency announcement is made in code language over the hospital P.A. system ("Code Red, Room 227," for example); this alarm alerts physicians and other specialists of an imminent death. Every available physician is then expected to rush to the bedside of the dying patient. Special emergency squads race through the halls, and the patient is hooked up to monitors and life-saving machinery which elicit a variety of visual and auditory signals. "It's a frantic, noisy, confused state," said one physician; "people in white clothing hurry about knocking themselves out to keep the patient alive." Not until every life-saving attempt has been exhausted do they let up. In the hospital setting, such extraordinary efforts to revive the patient and prolong life are routine.[12]

Although members of the medical staff rarely give verbal praise for a job well done, they are fiercely critical of haphazard clinical performance. Clinical pathology conferences, called CPCs or "death rounds," provide a forum for this expression. Whenever a patient dies, the residents, interns, attending staff, and others gather in an auditorium to discuss the "case." Whoever was responsible for the patient presents the clinical history and then the pathology report is given. Everyone then discusses what should have been done differently to avoid the death. "This gave me the idea," one physician said, "that if we were just smarter and had not made this or that mistake the patient would still be alive." Clearly, the assumption is that death is preventable and is not supposed to happen to good physicians. At least, this is the idea that is "handed down" to medical trainees. No wonder a sense of personal defeat is felt when patients die.

At this stage of training, then, death is viewed as the enemy, the opponent, something waiting to snatch away the patient. "The whole idea of medical training," said one physician, "is to teach doctors how to avoid death at almost any cost." So the battle lines are drawn, with death lurking in the shadows in mortal conflict with the physician, attired appropriately in white. At stake is not only the patient's life, but also the clinician's reputation and self-esteem.

Stage IV: Questioning the Medical Model[13]

With increasing experience, some clinicians begin to question and then to reject the prominent values espoused in medical training about death and dying.[14] The medical teaching model, as these physicians come to perceive it, tends to dehumanize the patient and to make a mere technician out of the doctor. That is, it glorifies the science of medicine (a thorough knowledge of disease processes and a ready command of clinical technique) at the expense of the art of medicine (an interpersonal ability to meet the patient's need by relating warmly and meaningfully to him and his family). In the physician's quest to master the science of medicine, he comes to regard the patient as an object or thing rather than as a fellow human being. "I hate to admit it," one physician reflected, "but I had come to view the patient almost as an extension of the apparatus in the room."

When death is viewed as the enemy, it is easy to overdo things, to go to extremes in prolonging life. "We would just go on forever," one confessed, "unless someone stopped us." Reflecting back, another physician came to the conclusion he had become so imbued with the idea of combating death that medical practice had become "a contest between me and the disease; the patient was merely an object over which we were fighting."

The turning point comes when those who reach this questioning stage can no longer escape the absurd extremes to which efforts are sometimes taken to keep patients alive. An intern, for example, was appalled by the efforts of his associates to prolong the life of a 17-year-old boy who had accidentally had part of his head shot off. Despite the fact that the boy had no cerebrum and was doomed to a vegetable-like existence, they wouldn't let him die. Instead, they kept him alive for several years, running up an enormous hospital and medical bill. Throughout all of this, his distraught mother daily put cream on his bedsores at a cost of $80 a bottle. "They were just prolonging a horrible state of affairs," he realized, "because nobody would accept the finality of it. It was kind of a personal failure to let him die."

One physician, who was an exemplary model of his former indoctrination, always worked fiercely to do his duty in combating death. On one occasion, for example, after an unsuccessful effort to resuscitate an elderly man, he became angry when the deceased patient's priest, who was waiting with the family in the adjoining room, acted as though death was a welcome blessing. Although the doctor said nothing at the time, he confessed, "I got angry as hell at him."

One day, though, a particularly harrowing experience "got to" him, and, in those brief hours, he came to question the values implicit in the medical model. For example, after 19 years of general practice, he admitted to the hospital an aging lady of about 75 with her fourth myocardial infarction. During the night she "died" five times and was resuscitated four. During the fourth resuscitation, the weary physician reflected on the "scene of wild chaos" and wondered, "What the hell are we doing to this poor lady? This is no way to die." He recalled, "Here was this little old lady lying spread-eagled across the bed with her tongue hanging out of one side of her mouth and a tube in the other and I thought to myself, 'Why?'" Then, answering his own question, he thought, "Because we haven't guts enough to stop, that's why." This conclusion was reinforced when for the fourth time he bore the news of resuscitation to the daughter who was waiting outside. Rather than thanking him for his heroic effort, the heartsick woman simply looked at him and, in a pleading voice, said "Please. . . ."

Such experiences stimulate some physicians to question whether their efforts to avoid death at any cost are really appropriate; and some eventually come to believe, as one said, that, in certain instances, people have "a right to die." "I have gotten beyond the stage concerned about technique and the notion that death implies failure," one practicing doctor said. "I've come to accept the fact that death is not the enemy, not something that must be conquered by the physician. People have a right to die in peace and dignity."

The extraordinary efforts to keep some patients functioning are seen by such doctors as "just so much medical pyrotechnics," designed to fulfill the physician's own needs rather than those of the patient and his family. One said, "The function of medical heroics is to demonstrate how good we are with our fancy gadgets; a good doctor can win recognition by keeping the poor old body going forever." In other words, professional recognition and self-esteem come to a physician by demonstrating technical ability (for instance, the ability to perform an appendectomy with only a buttonhole scar). But not much recognition comes from one's colleagues by being known as a warm and kind clinician who is compassionate and sympathetic.

A doctor's ego is easily inflated when he is cast in the role of the healer with power over death. When patients must entrust their lives to the physician, they naturally want to believe in his healing powers. Placed on a pedestal, he can easily feel omnipotent and become intoxicated with a sense of his own powers.[15] When his self-esteem is involved, it is imperative that he prevent death from occurring, for death makes him feel vulnerable. But if he can keep the "corpse" alive for a few more days or weeks, his mastery over death is demonstrated. "He's not about to let his omnipotence be challenged if he can help it," said one; "but if you talk to the family, you'll find that they are usually sorry that the patient had to suffer those extra days and that the hospital bill ran up so high."

As physicians at this stage view it, "the God complex" is incompatible with good medical practice. In their view it is unrealistic to expect a cure for everybody and inappropriate in many situations to unnecessarily prolong life. After all, death is, sooner or later, inevitable for everyone. In the final analysis, then, one cannot control death but can only temporarily delay it for shorter or longer periods, as the case may be. In this larger view the physician is, in reality, only a humble bystander.

Physicians who have reached this stage perceive a good clinician to be one who has mastered the art as well as the science of medicine, an achievement which was aptly summarized by the physician who said, "In the medical profession there are lots of doctors [i.e., techicians], but only relatively few physicians." It is the latter who, rather than possessing a compulsive concern for demonstrating clinical mastery over death, deem it imperative to consider the feelings of the patient and his family.

Stage V: Dealing with Personal Feelings

Up to this point their experience has conditioned clinicians to repress or suppress personal anxieties and fears about death. Everyone knows that the good doctor is supposed to be calm, with his own feelings under control—someone on whom the family can rely for steady support, insight, and understanding. The doctor who feels anxiety or fear in the face of death must carefully conceal these emotions. "I've had a lot of training in putting up a good front so that others can't see what I'm feeling inside," one said. "I've learned to keep this cool facade of being in control, but inside I'm feeling a lot of stress."

Our interviews with physicians revealed rather dramatically how much suppressed emotionality exists among medical practitioners. When probed, most of them disclosed unresolved psychic problems, some of which create severe stress. During our interviews, several wept. A research note by the interviewer indicates, "These interviews are getting markedly more difficult. Everybody I've talked to so far is having a horrible time dealing with death and dying; and it isn't just on a professional level, but personally, too." Surprisingly, one physician unmasked a phobia of death. "I'm really horrified by looking at or being near dead bodies," he said. Throughout medical training and practice, this physician had tried to avoid the presence of corpses but, of course, this was not always possible. So he had experienced some extremely stressful times, as one might imagine.

His phobia stemmed from a childhood experience at the funeral of his father, a scene which has lingered with him through the years.

> I walked up to the coffin and was startled by this awful, mottled, purple-looking face. They hadn't done a very good job of preserving and embalming him. After all of these years I still wake up at night and am actually scared to open my eyes because I can see my father—the dead figure—standing in a corner. I tell myself, "Hey, you're being silly," but I haven't got rid of it yet.

Tragically, not once during the entire period of this troubled physician's medical training did any mentor provide an opportunity for him to ventilate his fears and anxieties. Although he has developed ample technical skills and is now recognized as an accomplished physician, he is, in part, by his own admission, emotionally crippled.

Other physicians, too, revealed anxieties related to the personal loss of loved ones, the sense of helplessness in dealing with hopeless diseases, and the disquieting experience of inadvertently "killing" a patient through error or bad advice. For instance, one physician, while yet an intern, had this traumatic experience:

> A woman came in with severe ascites and I did a paracentesis on her. As we were getting the fluid she went into shock and died. At the "post" we found that the trochar had gone through an

aberrant major artery in the abdominal wall. This shook me up
pretty badly. Although it wasn't done deliberately, I had actually
killed somebody. I felt very upset!

Although his technical procedures were critically reviewed in the
death conference, no one gave the heartsick doctor any help with
regard to his emotions. Instead, like other medical trainees, he was
left to work out his feelings on his own.

Until physicians reach this stage of self-examination, they often
cope with impending death by utilizing avoidance as a technique. "I
try to keep away from patients if I know what's coming up so as to
reduce the emotional stress," a medical student confessed. Feelings
of helplessness stimulated by hopelessly ill patients can be relieved
by passing these patients off to someone else or by being too busy to
spend much time with them. When contact must be made by the
physician, he can simply check the equipment, write the orders and
say, "Hi! How are you feeling?" then bustle off to see someone else.[16]
"We ignore the patient because we are so fearful ourselves," one
commented.[17]

Typically every effort is made in the hospital setting to shield
oneself from mourning relatives. In the emergency room quiet crying
is tolerated, but if any kind of emotional outburst occurs, relatives
are usually hustled off to the chapel as fast as possible. "We isolate
them so that their grief is not so obvious," a physican said. "It isn't
done cruelly, but, frankly, it is done more to protect the emergency
room staff than to help the family."

The physician transcends this stage of avoidance as he begins to
realize that how one feels inside is much more important than what
is actually being said and done. Self-examination is stimulated when,
in trying to be more than a mere technician, he tries to deal
meaningfully with the feelings of patients and their families. If he is
truly to assist others in more than a technical sense, a doctor must
come to grips with his own feelings. How can he allay others' fears
and anxieties if he denies the inevitability of death or fails to
acknowledge his own mortality? Is it realistic to expect comforting
relief from one who in his own training has had such little supportive
help in dealing with his own feelings?

Reflecting back upon their earlier training, physicians at this
stage fault their mentors for giving them such little help with the
subjective aspects of death. "It's almost as though I've had to deal
with this part of medical practice without being prepared for it," one
said. "In most every other aspect of my training, I've had a chance to
observe my preceptors and then discuss the experience." On the

topic of death, however, medical trainees are left to their own common sense assumptions. The few who were fortunate enough to receive some instruction on this topic characterized the pedagogical experience as being intellectualized and abstract. The topic of how to handle a dying patient was dealt with, one said, "in cookbook-like fashion, no different than if we were learning to work up a case of hypertension." Another pointed out, "We were never asked to express our feelings or discuss how we felt about death." Nor could any physician recall a single experience where a clinical mentor openly revealed his own feelings about death—the frustrations, anger, or feelings of hopelessness that occur when a patient dies. So each medical trainee is left to his own resources in resolving inner dilemmas on this sensitive subject.

The result of this unhappy state of affairs is, as has been indicated, that until he does come to grips with his feelings, the doctor tends to depersonalize the patient or, failing that, to avoid him and his family. And, as previously mentioned, the system of recognition and rewards which operates in the medical milieu reinforces the tendency to be analytical and nonemotional. "I can speak for myself and possibly for a lot of other physicians," one practicing doctor said. "In my younger years my professional self-image wouldn't permit me to be slowed down or have my efficiency reduced by my feelings. So I evolved into a condition of what I now call 'disembodied intelligence.' But now I'm trying to get more and more in touch with my own feelings, to recognize and tolerate them, and thereby be in a better position to help others with their feelings."

Once having reached this stage, the introspective physician who has recognized his own feelings and limitations, and has managed to reconcile them as well, is uniquely capable of practicing compleat medicine. He alone has the personal ability and resources to bring technical knowledge and sympathetic care to dying patients and their loved ones.

CONCLUSION

The career path to physicianhood is a well-marked route. One begins as a freshman medical student and then advances to successive stages of sophomore, junior, and then senior. After medical school graduation, the fledgling doctor becomes an intern, then a resident, and, finally, a private practitioner.[18] During this long journey, medical aspirants undergo a variety of personally challenging experiences, not the least of which is dealing with dying patients and their families.[9]

At the journey's outset medical recruits are no better prepared for dealing with death than their contemporaries, and initially they respond as laymen. Inexperienced and idealistic, many become disillusioned, with about one in ten dropping out, mostly during the first year. Those who press foreward must develop emotional callouses; they must become accustomed to dealing with stressful circumstances, such as death, which normally are upsetting. The fact that their patients expect them to be sympathetic and compassionate, as well as technically competent, is no small challenge. Yet the development and maintenance of this delicate balance is the test of true skill in fulfilling the physician's role.

Longitudinal observations make clear the social processes which condition rookie clinicians to handle death and dying with rationality and composure. However, the educational processes which foster empathy and compassion are not clearly visible. Death is a daily occurrence in the teaching hospital, but talk about death as a stressful human vicissitude is almost nonexistent.

Medical educators seem no less inhibited in their ability to verbalize feelings about death than the lay public.[20] As the socializing system now operates, if a medical journeyman is to come to grips with his own feelings so that he can interact comfortably with dying patients in this awesome yet ubiquitous experience, he must do it on his own. Unfortunately this self-analysis does not always happen to those who travel the career pathway.[21]

La Rochefoucauld has said, "One cannot look directly at either the sun or death" (Lifton and Olson, 1974). Due to this human frailty, a wall of silence often surrounds the dying patient at a time when feelings cry for expression. The very facts from which the patient is usually shielded are the same ones that he is forced to live and die with, and quite alone.[22] As commander-in-chief at the death scene, an event which now typically occurs in hospitals and extended care settings rather than in the familiar setting of one's own home, the physician has great potential for rendering healing aid in a spiritual or humanistic as well as a technical sense. The doctor is in a unique position to ease the fear, alienation, and loneliness of the dying patient. But if his mastery of the healing arts includes only an ability to patch up and keep the body functioning, he leaves unfulfilled the yearnings of the human soul at one of life's most dramatic and important moments.[23]

The developmental personality changes which result from medical socialization, as now constituted, are not conducive to preparing the doctor emotionally so that he can meet the needs of dying patients and their families in the depersonalized hospital setting. Little recognition currently exists among medical educators that the doctor's role is more than that of gatekeeper of the nation's health—that, in fact, he also presides over the death scene.[24] If he is to fulfill the role which is increasingly expected of him, he must be better prepared to deal with the subjective features of this poignant experience.

NOTES

1. For background information concerning the cultural roots of death orientations in American society, see Parsons and Lidz (1967).

2. For a discussion of the competing demands inherent in the doctor's role, see Merton (1957), especially pp. 73–79.

3. The topic of death and dying was but one of many covered during the interviews, which varied in length from 1.5 to 3 hours, depending on student loquatiousness. More than 200 items of information were included in the recorded questions and answers. Results of the larger study will soon be published in a book entitled *Students into Doctors: Professional Socialization in Medical School* (by R. H. Coombs, in preparation).

4. Interviews were conducted on the West Coast before Dr. Powers accepted her present position. The 13 physicians interviewed ranged in age from 30 to 57, with a mean age of 41. Three were women, ten were men, and all but one, an anesthesiologist, were currently in psychiatric training or in the private practice of psychiatry. The physicians interviewed have a wide variety of experience. Eight were in general practice prior to beginning psychiatric training; among these the average length of general practice was 12 years, with a range of from 2 to 25 years. One physician interviewed had been an anesthesiologist for 7 years. Two physicans who took part in the study had been in the service after internship and prior to psychiatric training. The two physicians remaining had gone directly through psychiatric training. One of the physicians was a minister and one was a social worker prior to going to medical school. Ten of the 13 physicians interviewed went to medical school in the United States, and three were trained in foreign countries.

5. A further discussion on the topic of the medical center as a social system is given by Bloom (1971).

6. An earlier report about the coping mechanisms utilized by seasoned clinicians in stressful hospital situations is provided in Coombs and Goldman (1973). This research, part of the larger study of medical socialization, was based upon participant observation in an intensive care unit.

7. Kasper (1959) first emphasized that medical students are desensitized not to death, but to the symbols of death.

8. For further discussion on this and other aspects of the desensitizing experience, see Lief and Fox's (1963) article.

9. Humor is also utilized as a tension release in subsequent stages of professional development. Lightheartedness in the midst of painful human drama might seem inappropriate, but it helps to reduce the emotional tension and strain created by stressful circumstances and thereby allows clinicians to perform their responsibilities more effectively.

10. The whole tone of the autopsy room differs from the clinical cadaver setting. There is only one body (instead of several lined up in rows), and it has not been chemically treated in any way as have the cadavers, so it is much easier to perceive it as a live person. Also, the attending physician is nearly always present (rather than anatomy instructors), and this helps define the dead person as a patient rather than a specimen.

11. Students rarely have an opportunity to follow a patient longitudinally, since their clinical assignments include frequent rotations from one clinical service to another. This shuttling back and forth from one hospital setting to another usually does not allow them enough time to form close personal attachments with patients.

12. For further reading on the social organization related to death in the hospital setting, see Sudnow (1967).

13. By the term "medical model," we mean primarily that system of clinical practice which exists in American teaching hospitals, one which includes a technological emphasis tending to exclude the humanistic dimensions of medical practice.

14. It is our impression that most clinicians who reach this questioning stage do so after graduating from medical school. But some clinical medical students are aware of the critical views of more advanced physicians. "I've heard that no one dies with dignity in this hospital," one said, "There is always a crowd of people around frantically working over him and hooking him up to gadgets."

15. In this regard, Mace (1971) has said, "If I may coin a word, I would suggest that the medical disease of today is 'pedestalitis.' The doctor is on a pedestal, and his elevation is to some extent gratifying; but it also makes him feel isolated, cut off, and somewhat insecure. ... More and more he is seen as an authority figure, a busy human dynamo, who is not to be bothered with little human concerns and does not have time to sit down and talk. He is remote and detached, like the man who sits at the controls in the lonely box that operates a giant crane."

16. Technical jargon also helps avoid the stressful dialogue with patients and their families. These terms tend to isolate death by classifying it as a medical event—an event occurring in professional life rather than personal life. For further discussion about language as a coping mechanism, see Coombs and Goldman (1973).

17. There is evidence, too, that patients sometimes help doctors avoid the discomfort of talking about death by not asking questions or pressing for details. This reinforces the commonly held assumption that terminal patients do not want to talk about death.

18. Of course, those who become general practitioners avoid the residency stage. Also, internship has been eliminated in the training of some specialties.

19. For an interesting essay on the doctor and his training, see chapter 2, "The Man Behind the Stethoscope," in Greenberg (1965).

20. Glaser and Strauss (1968) have said, "The psychological aspects of dealing with the dying and their families are virtually absent from training. Hence, although physicians and nurses are highly skilled at handling the bodies of terminal patients, their behavior to them otherwise is actually outside the province of professional standards."

21. In other words, Stage V could come earlier and with much greater ease if

medical educators would recognize and openly discuss with trainees their feelings about death and dying.

22. Recognizing this unmet human need, commercial agencies have sprung up to provide, for a fee, companions for those dying of incurable diseases. According to a UPI dispatch (*Star Free Press*, Ventura, California, February 27, 1975), this new service appears to be a lucrative business.

23. Kübler-Ross (1969) maintains that ours is the most death-denying society of all time. Because death has traditionally been a taboo subject, relatively little has been written on the topic. Quite recently, however, an increasing number of books and articles have been written and seminars initiated on the new subject—"Thanatology, the study of death"—in colleges and medical schools.

24. We suspect, however, that there will be significant changes in the coming years. Research by Kübler-Ross and others has piqued interest and awareness of the problem. Most interesting are the development of health-care organizations, like the New Haven Hospices, which furnish doctors and paramedics to monitor the dying patient and look after his welfare, counsel the family, and provide emotional support (Dobihal, 1974).

REFERENCES

Bloom, S.W. (1971) "The medical center as a social system," pp. 429–448 in R. H. Coombs and C. E. Vincent (eds.) Psychosocial Aspects of Medical Training. Springfield, Ill.: Charles C Thomas.

Coombs, R. H. and L. J. Goldman (1973) "Maintenance and discontinuity of coping mechanisms in an intensive-care unit." Social Problems 20 (Winter): 342–355.

Dobihal, E. F., Jr. (1974) "Talk on terminal care." Connecticut Medicine 38 (July): 364–367.

Glaser, B. G. and A. L. Strauss (1968) A Time for Dying. Chicago: Aldine.

Greenberg, S. (1965) The Troubled Calling: Crisis in the Medical Establishment. New York: Macmillan.

Kasper, A. M. (1959) "The doctor and death," pp. 259–271 in H. Feifel (ed.) The Meaning of Death, New York: McGraw-Hill.

Kübler-Ross, E. (1969) On Death and Dying. New York: Macmillan.

Lief, H. I. and R. C. Fox (1963) "The medical student's training for 'detached concern,'" pp. 12–35 in H. I. Lief, V. Lief and N. R. Lief (eds.) The Psychological Basis of Medical Practice. New York: Harper & Row.

Lifton, R. J. and E. Olson (1974) Living and Dying. New York: Praeger.

Mace, D. R. (1971) "Communication, interviewing, and the physician-patient relationship," pp. 380–403 in R. H. Coombs and C. E. Vincent (eds.) Psychosocial Aspects of Medical Training. Springfield, Ill.: Charles C Thomas.

Merton, R. K. (1957) "Some preliminaries to a sociology of medical education," pp. 3–79 in R. K. Merton, G. Reader and P. L. Kendall (eds.) The Student-Physician: Introductory Studies in the Sociology of Medical Education. Cambridge, Mass.: Harvard Univ. Press.

Parsons, T. and V. Lidz (1967) "Death in American society," pp. 133–170 in E. S. Schneidman (ed.) Essays in Self-Destruction. New York: Science House.

Sudnow, D. (1967) Passing On: The Social Organization of Dying. Englewood Cliffs, N.J.: Prentice-Hall.

On My Medical Education:
Seeking a Balance in Medicine

Scott May

I perceive there to be a serious imbalance not only in medical education but also in most institutions of technologically developed countries. There are many ways to characterize this imbalance. The opposing forces involved can be viewed from varying systems. I hope that at least one of these dichotomies will sound familiar: mechanical over humanistic; objective over subjective; yang over yin; thinking over feeling; efficiency over creativity; animus over anima; John Wayne over Sophia Loren; the male principles over the female principles.

For convenience I use the terms male principles and female principles to encompass the two sides of this situation, but in so doing I do not wish to imply that only males have male principles operating or that only females have female principles operating. In fact, I will attempt to demonstrate that all men and women have varying proportions of both principles operating and it is only for purposes of illustration that I have chosen to use this historical and mythological classification of character traits. Under the rubric of male principles I include competition, aggression, logic, striving, objectifying, intellect, and power. Under the banner of the female principles I include relatedness, receptivity, creativity, sensitivity, subjectivity, feeling and nurturance. I will try to illustrate how this relative preponderance of male principles and the relative absence of female principles operates in medical education, what its consequences are for both patients and for physicians, and some suggestions on ways that it might be rebalanced.

First, I would like to establish the fact that I value, in fact highly value, the technological, logical, and tough-minded training that I have acquired in medical school. I am a strong believer in the importance of discipline, responsibility, the taking on of challenges, striving for excellence and even for power in most endeavors, including medicine. In many ways, these male principles were the ones that enabled me to get into medical school and that I had come to hold in high regard. My appreciation for these male principles was demonstrated to me more vividly than I could have envisioned last weekend while working on this speech. I was returning to San Francisco from Stinson Beach when I came upon a serious car accident where one of the passengers was trapped underneath the car, unconscious and bleeding profusely from his mouth. Four years ago I would have known enough to call an ambulance and hope for a doctor to come; this time I was the doctor—using CPR, starting I.V.'s, injecting Bicarb, suctioning. At that moment I was all action and fast thinking, hallmarks of the male principle. There was neither time nor room for feelings as I put my mouth over this man's broken, blood-filled mandible.

Medicine, however, is not a succession of traumatic emergencies and code blues. It is not a battlefield where one can claim that a creative, feeling, and sensitive person only gets in the way. On the contrary, medicine is composed primarily of small human stories involving souls and feelings as well as bodies that need balancing and nurturance. Medicine needs the female principles, the yin side of life, just as it needs the male principles, the yang side of life. The public is asking for compassion, nurturance, and sensitivity as well as competence, intelligence, and dedication from their physicians. Too much of anything, no matter how intrinsically good it may seem, is damaging—be it water in water intoxication, strawberry jam, or the male principle of endless striving for perfection at almost any cost.

While I am grateful for knowing what to do in a medical emergency, the acquisition of that knowledge and many other skills deriving from male principles in medicine came at an enormous and what I feel to be excessive and possibly even destructive cost. The reason that it feels so costly is that in the process of learning and incorporating this medical knowledge, there was tremendous institutional pressure to ignore, devalue, and even disown my own female principles. Nurturance, tenderness, and soulfulness were being crowded out by perfection, evaluation, and the demand for performance.

Several students from my class were concerned enough that at the end of their second year of medical school they asked the dean's office to do a survey of students' changes in self-concept during medical school. The findings are as follows:

The majority of respondents describe themselves as having been intellectually honest, competent, organized, calm, enthusiastic, and happy most of the time before entering medical school. After two years of medical school, more than half of the respondents described themselves as less creative and more pressured and coerced than previously, although two thirds continued to see themselves as intellectually honest. At the same time, thirty-eight to forty-eight percent reported that they perceived themselves as less competent, more demoralized, more angry, more confused, more anxious, more depressed, and more ambivalent than before.

The damaging consequences of this abundance of male principles and paucity of female principles in medicine is not limited just to medical students. It seems that the proliferation of malpractice suits as well as the seeking out by intelligent people of unconventional healers and quacks is a rebellion against the reliance on solely technological rather than a balance of humanistic and technological means of physicians' relating to their patients. The public is beginning to seek out practitioners who have mastered the female principles as they relate to healing. Because of their previous disenchantment with predominantly technologically oriented physicians, the public has become less discriminating about evaluating a practitioner's mastery of the male principles of healing when selecting a healer. I do not mean to imply that there are no physicians who have incorporated both principles in balanced amounts. They do exist. I have worked with several here at U.C. They are the physicians sought out by medical students and patients alike, again and again.

In order for the female principles to develop and to come close to balancing the male principles, they need to be respected and nurtured. They are subtler and less tangible than the products deriving from male principle endeavors. As scientists we often have difficulty with this fact. Medical school, instead of rebalancing this equation, has increased the imbalance each year—frequently treating the people and situations exhibiting female principles in a harsh, often deprecating, fashion, while often glorifying the male principles. Medical school felt like a family where the mother was gone and only the hard father remained at home. I and many of my classmates experienced this imbalance in a multitude of ways under varying conditions. I have selected a group of experiences from my four years of medical school to try to illustrate how this imbalance is perpetuated.

1. In the pursuit of the male principles of sacrifice and deprivation, most of my classmates will undoubtably remember a particular biochemistry lecturer who upon learning that the majority of our class had not read his syllabus before the lecture launched into

a monologue extolling the virtues of beginning our sleep deprivation now rather than waiting for our clinical years. He exhorted us to read the syllabus no matter what the hour, urging us for the sake of science to push ourselves harder while ignoring messages from the very bodies we were studying.

2. As an example of taking a male principle like efficiency to such an extreme that the original reason is lost, one only has to think of the practice of excluding fathers from the delivery room because they might get in the way or contaminate the field. Yet who is going to be taking care of that baby? What does the mother want? Who is taking responsibility for infant–parent bonding? And how many sterile vaginal deliveries have any of us really witnessed? Another example of efficiency dominating feeling was the policy until recently of limiting the visiting hours of parents on pediatric floors. Surely it can be a nuisance to have someone asking questions while changing an I.V. bottle in a child's room, but who stands the best chance of diminishing the trauma and anxiety of a hospitalization for a child?

3. In a seemingly well-motivated desire to be as objective and scientific as possible, certainly respectable male principles, we lose sight of who we are really helping, of the subjective side of our patients. How many patients do we all remember because of their disease, their pathology, their physical presentation, and possibly their face? We don't remember their names or who they live with. We don't know or remember what is really important to each of them. Yet what is the patient feeling and thinking? What do they remember about themselves? Do they think of themselves as aortic aneurysms or papilledema? How many times in my preclinical years did I hear lip service about the importance of obtaining a good social history on a patient compared to the number of times my attending urged me to speed through to the pertinent positives and negatives, and to dispense with the social history? I am familiar with the argument that this objectification of the patient is necessary for professional distance. What purpose does this distance serve? I feel that it is invoked as a necessary practice much the same way the Pentagon stamps everything top secret. Certainly objectification has its place in medicine. I believe it makes sense to drape a patient during surgery so one can concentrate on the tissue. I also believe that during the ride down the elevator to the operating room and for those few minutes before the patient is anesthetized, he needs warmth, real contact, and concern more than almost any time during his hospital stay. Yet who usually accompanies him at this time—another unknown face.

4. The annihilation of feelings and sensitivity through fatigue and the glorification of a rigorous, tough, superhuman call schedule

seems to lead in one of two directions. If we become inefficient and slightly fuzzy-headed after thirty straight hours of work, we feel we have failed to measure up to the standards of medicine. If on the other hand, we succeed in driving ourselves, keeping our perform-ance up to snuff, then we begin to see ourselves as a separate breed, superior to the rest of mankind. This display of superhuman endurance, an example of a male principle, ultimately manifests as contempt for those patients who complain about their life and troubles on a cushy eight hours of sleep. In some of us it leads to arrogance, one of the cardinal signs of male principle excess. How is it that we praise those interns who elect an every other night rotation rather than question their priorities and the emptiness in the rest of their lives?

5. While doing the infamous extremity service out at San Francisco General Hospital I had an experience which demonstrated a contempt for tenderness and the familiar dynamic of the oppressed identifying with and eventually exhibiting the behavior of the oppressor. I was trying to talk down an I.V. drug user who was being put under general anesthesia for an I & D (incision and drainage) that I was about to perform. The patient was a nervous, difficult person, but he was slowly calming down. In the midst of this, a seemingly reasonable, decent anesthesia resident yelled at me to shut up and to get out of the way and to quit letting myself be manipulated by this addict. I couldn't help but wonder why the resident had come to feel that compassion, even compassion being manipulated, was so distasteful. It seemed that he had had that female principle driven out of him and he didn't like being reminded of that fact.

6. My last category of ward experiences that illustrate the reinforcement of male principles at the expense of female principles is the take-home message for most medical students and house officers that it is one's performance that counts, not one's feelings. Last year, a good friend of mine—a neurology resident at Stanford—shot himself in the head. None of his colleagues saw it coming. Is it any surprise, given the enormous responsibilities and demands and the few established or respected means of expressing the difficulty this brings, that more than one hundred physicians kill themselves and over three hundred physicians become addicted to Demerol every year? This is equivalent to three of our graduating medical school classes each year and it does not take into account the new alcoholics, divorces, or severe mental illnesses.

7. In contrast to the examples I just mentioned, there were times when female principles were operating in harmony and on equal footing with male principles in medical school. The moments that

stand out to me include several sets of attending rounds where I was impressed by the attending physician's sensitivity and discretion with particular patients; a team celebration with a patient who was leaving the hospital after six weeks of a series of life-threatening conditions; my junior surgery team when we xeroxed articles for each other, took notes for each other, and laughed a great deal while working hard; the genuine feelings one could sense at the funeral this year of one of my classmates who had such a wonderful blend of the male and female principles in her life; and the wisdom of U.C.S.F. to do away with grades and class ranking, putting cooperation ahead of competition without losing high quality.

I know it is possible, therefore, to create situations where female principles are given more prominence and respect, but it will not happen without a conscious effort from all of us. Unless more than the current level of lip service is used to rectify this imbalance, the explosion of scientific information, the accelerating demand for services, the expansion of health technologies, and the more intense competition for prized professional positions and grants will further distort the imbalance toward the male principles.

I have some general suggestions that I feel will help to rebalance the situation and make for more whole physicians. I also have some specific thoughts for my classmates, the faculty, and the alumni.

In order to allow house officers enough time to respond to all of their patients and to medical students, the patient load and hence the teaching material may have to be reduced. In order to allow house officers to spend time revitalizing their lives, their call schedules may have to be reduced or there may have to be a special night call established which would mean that everyone would see fewer "great cases," but they would remember those cases they did participate in without bitterness or fatigue.

It would mean spending faculty time overseeing the well-being as well as the didactic instruction of medical students, hence taking some time away from pure academic teaching. It would also mean establishing priorities that emphasized the attainment of balance rather than perfection, which might make for lower national board scores but longer-living physicians. It might require the chairmen of departments and the senior faculty taking the unpleasant step of reprimanding those faculty members and house officers found abusing or intimidating students, other house officers, or patients, and making it clear that this is unacceptable behavior regardless of how brilliant one might be. It would encourage faculty and house officers to value rather than deprecate those students who are less thick-skinned and less distant from their own feelings and those of the patients, and to look for them on the admissions committee.

Specifically for my classmates, I urge you to remember your heart—not to separate your feelings from your thoughts so far that you cannot easily reunite them. Demand the right to be treated warmly and genuinely, and demand the time required to respond to your family, your friends, and your patients in a similar manner.

To the faculty and alumni, I encourage you to consider what I have just said to my classmates and I would also like to remind you that you are the people who set the tone. The questions you ask, the feedback you give, the emphasis you present can tip this male principles/female principles equation in either direction. It takes just one of you with a balanced approach to keep a student believing a balance is possible. If you feel that the female principles elude you or that they are not part of your style you can still restrain yourself and your colleagues from undermining those who are trying to incorporate both into a meaningful way to practice medicine; and you can go out of your way to encourage those students who are still trying for the best of both worlds.

We can all look forward to a time when another medical student stands up here and asks for more time for the male principles.

Rebelling Against Big Brother

Mark B. Wenneker

Remember those first days of medical school in Amphitheater C? As we gazed over the eager faces, we all knew who would become the surgeons, the researchers, and the family practitioners. Did any of us suspect then that our class would produce eight anesthesiologists, 10 radiologists, 14 ophthalmologists, and one of the lowest percentages of general internists and surgeons in the history of Harvard Medical School? I certainly didn't. What makes us so different? Maybe it's the $30,000 debt that many of us have incurred, but surely business school was an easier way to make a buck. I think that behind these statistics lies a deeper meaning about how we wish to incorporate medicine into our lives.

There was a time in the not-so-distant past when graduation from medical school was like a marriage ceremony. Our medical forefathers (we have few foremothers) took their vows to devote their lives to medicine, for better or for worse, for richer or for . . . well, till death did they part. Residents—as the word suggests—*resided* in the hospital. Salaries were minimal, but who needed money when food and clothes were free and one didn't need an accountant to calculate a debt repayment schedule? There was even a time when hospitals forbade their residents to marry. After all, that would be bigamy.

Some may say that times have changed. Yet, a few months ago as I was flipping through the pages of the *Boston Globe*, I happened upon Ann Landers' column, which included a letter from a "concerned mother" whose son, Jay, was an intern under stress. Poor Jay was so exhausted that he could no longer make clinical decisions. Worse, his mother was terribly worried. Knowing how fair and open-minded Ann is, I looked forward to a gentle but scathing critique of the medical training process and a discussion of the importance of a balanced life. Instead, she turned to a surgeon friend from Stanford for the definitive answer. He was far from sympathetic. Without qualification he asserted that "young doctors, in order to gain as much clinical experience as possible, would rather take care of patients than either eat or sleep." And I thought Stanford was laid-back! He went on to say that the "real shakers and movers in medicine are those with total commitment." In other words, "Sorry, Mom, Jay's just a wimp."

As a member of the Harvard family, I have heard again and again that I will be a future leader of medicine, a shaker and a mover. Nobody ever told me that being a leader meant preferring the care of patients to eating or sleeping, not to mention other enjoyable pastimes.

I ask my classmates. "How many of you want to be shakers and movers? And at what cost?" Most of us are not here today to take marriage vows. We were admitted to HMS because of our diversity of interests. Some of us were musicians, others journalists, many brilliant scientists; each was unique. The theme of our second-year show was that we wanted to maintain that uniqueness. The career decisions of the Class of 1984 are messages to Big Brother, at Stanford or anywhere else, that our careers will not consume our lives.

To some of you, our views might be heresy. But today fewer physicians are willing to make a total commitment to their careers. Once doctors were idolized for their devotion to their patients, but the age of the medical hero is passing. As medicine has become more esoteric and technology more complex, doctors have distanced themselves from their patients. The traditional question, "Is this the best treatment for my patient?" no longer suffices in the face of health-care budget restraints. When prescribing a liver transplant, we are forced to look beyond the patient's interest and consider the cost to society. Being a hero isn't as easy as it once was. Medical malpractice and a more aware public have reduced doctors from gods to mere mortals.

Until recently, few doctors would admit that total commitment had its personal cost. Yet the rates of suicide, alcoholism, and drug abuse among physicians—up to eight times higher, maybe more, than among the general population—attest to the toll stress takes on our lives. A recent *JAMA* article found the major source of dissatisfaction among primary care practitioners to be "too many patients to see in too short a time, too large a case load and too much time on call."

All of us need time for our families. More young doctors, male and female, want to play an active role in child rearing and not abdicate that responsibility to their respective partners. We want to be more than just good doctors, we want to be good parents and spouses as well.

Will medical care suffer? That's doubtful. David Fraser '69, president of Swarthmore College, asserts that physicians are much more useful to their patients if they have allowed themselves to develop fully. There are already signs of structural changes in health care that will enable physicians to accommodate a more balanced life. The explosion of HMOs and group practices offers us good salaries and reasonable working hours. And believe it or not, even residency programs have responded to pressure by house staff for more humane working conditions.

Can we still be shakers and movers? I believe the answer is yes. But, whatever gains we make in medicine, we will not lose sight of our other priorities. At the very least, I trust we will be competent physicians with meaningful lives. I wish the Class of 1984 the best of luck.

RECOMMENDED READING

Collins, Frances S., Ney, Robert L., Hadler, Norman M., McMillan, Campbell W., and Mangana, Charles, 1977, "The Medical Dilemma: Professional Demands and Personal Needs—A Panel Discussion," *The Pharos*, April Issue, 1978, pp. 29–34.

Coombs, Robert H., and Fawzy, Fawzy I., 1982, "The Effect of Marital Status on Stress in Medical School," *American Journal of Psychiatry*, Vol. 139, No. 11, pp. 1490–1493.

Coombs, Robert H., and Fawzy, Fawzy I., 1982, "Medical Marriage as Preventive for Physician Impairment," *California Academy of Family Practitioners*, Vol. 33, No. 4, pp. 14–18.

Fawzy, Fawzy I., Coombs, Robert H., and Wolcott, Deane L., in press, "Marital Status and Life Stress: A Literature Review," *Psychiatric Annals*.

Hundert, Edward M., 1984, "Medicine, Consistency and the Golden Rule," *Harvard Medical Alumni Bulletin*, Vol. 58, No. 3, pp. 18–19.

Nelson, Bryce, 1983, "Can Doctors Learn Warmth? Concern Over Lack of Compassion Leads to Nationwide Action." *The New York Times*, September 13, III, 1:4.

Ramen, Naomi, 1977, "Humanistic Medicine: Professionalism," *The New Physician*, Vol. 26, No. 11, pp. 45–46.

Samuels, Martin, 1984, "Requiem for Clarinet," *Harvard Medical Alumni Bulletin*, Vol. 58, No. 3, pp. 16–18.

Stone, John H., 1981, "Characteristics of the Compleat Physician," *The Pharos*, Fall Issue, pp. 16–20.

Verby, John E., 1980, "Equity and Balance," *Journal of Medical Education*, Vol. 55, November Issue, p. 981.

Index

About the Editors

Robert H. Coombs, Ph.D., is Professor of Biobehavioral Sciences (Medical Sociology) at UCLA School of Medicine and Director, Office of Education, UCLA Neuropsychiatric Institute and Hospital. His related books include *Psychosocial Aspects of Medical Training* (with C. E. Vincent; Thomas); *Mastering Medicine: Professional Socialization in Medical School* (The Free Press); and *Making It In Medical School* (with J. St. John; Medicine and Society Press/Peterson's Guides). He is a member of the Student Affairs Committee at UCLA School of Medicine and has offered courses for medical and premedical students and medical couples on the processes and outcomes of professional socialization in the medical career.

D.Scott May, M.D., is a National Institute of Mental Health Research Fellow and Assistant Clinical Professor of Psychiatry, UCLA School of Medicine. He received his medical training at the University of California, San Francisco, and at Stanford University. He has served on the National Committee on Residency for the American Psychiatrist Association and the Well Being Committees at UCSF, Stanford, and UCLA School of Medicine. He also counsels medical students with psychological problems.

Gary W. Small, M.D., is Assistant Professor of Psychiatry at the UCLA School of Medicine and a recipient of a Clinical Investigator Award from the National Institute on Aging. He was a Clinical Fellow in Psychiatry at Harvard Medical School and Chief Resident of the Psychiatric Consultation Service at Massachusetts General Hospital. He has taught premedical students on professional socialization in medicine and has led support groups for medical residents at both the UCLA Medical Center and Harvard Medical School.